YOU TAKE MY BREATH AWAY

BIKER BOB & AMIE KOSBERG

ISBN: 979-8-9858562-1-7 (Paperback)
     979-8-9858562-0-0 (Hardcover)
     979-8-9858562-2-4 (eBook)

Interior design by Booknook.biz

Table of Contents

Mission Statement

WE WROTE THIS BOOK TO RAISE AWARENESS of the plight of our environment with its pervasion of 350,000 synthetic chemicals that threaten humanity's existence and their effect on a personal level. We want to encourage more people to ask questions about the profusion of fragrances and chemicals that wreak havoc on millions of daily lives, and that are more and more often being blamed for illness and discomfort in many domains. We want the reader and the consumer to be aware of the negligence of companies and the government to protect individuals, society, and the planet.

This is a struggle that has been repeated many times: Agent Orange, asbestos, DDT, lead paint, and cigarette smoke have all caused death and suffering when profit is venerated above empathy. But truth tellers, activists and scientists enter the fray and demand justice. This book is our story and yours. It is time to leave behind stubbornness and replace it with knowledge and demand legislative action.

Opening Quotes

"32.2% OF ADULTS [THAT EQUATES to over 100+ million people] report fragrance sensitivity; that is, adverse health effects from fragranced consumer products, out of the 26% of the population that reports asthma/asthma-like conditions, 42.6% report chemical sensitivity and 57.8% report fragrance sensitivity." Anne Steinemann, "International prevalence of fragrance sensitivity," Springer Link June 1, 2019.

"Once thought to be safe, there is mounting evidence that human exposure to chemicals at low levels can be harmful." Nicholas A. Ashford and Claudia S. Miller, Environmental Science & Technology/News; 509A, November 1, 1998

"Emissions and exposures from fragranced consumer products, such as air fresheners and cleaning supplies, have been associated with health problems and societal impacts." Bridges, B. (2002). Fragrance: emerging health and environmental concerns. *Flavour and Fragrance Journal*, 17(5). 361-371.

"Fragrance chemicals are known to act as haptens in the skin and bind with body proteins to form allergens." Bridges, B.

"Asthma rates have soared since the 1970s. Fragrances and formaldehyde trigger and exacerbate asthma." Bridges, B.

"Fragrance can impact the brain and nervous system. Some of these effects are immediate and transitory, while others can be long-term. Olfactory pathways provide the most direct connection to the brain of any senses and also provide a means of toxic materials entering the brain." Bridges, B.

"Those that use scented products on a regular basis may not be able to detect their own fragrance shortly after applying it. They may apply increasing amounts or reapply frequently so that they can smell the fragrance. In many instances they are totally oblivious to the fact that their fragrance is often overwhelming and intrusive to others." Bridges, B.

"...Nerve poisons, called neurotoxins, are one of the leading causes of illness in the workplace. Daily exposure to neurotoxins can cause... disorders of the mind and body" ... and "can lead to irreversible disabling disorders that affect every aspect of a victim's life." Harold L. Volkmer, "Neurotoxins at home and in the workplace" House of Representatives, Committee on Science and Technology, October 8, 1985

"Those at greatest risk include the unborn or newborn child whose brain is inadequately shielded from toxic substances in the blood." Dr. Peter S. Spencer, Director, Institute of

Neurotoxicology, Albert Einstein College of Medicine, Bronx, NY, House of Representatives, Committee on Science and Technology, October 8, 1985

"Chemical pollution has passed safe limit for humanity…" *The Guardian* January 18, 2022

"350,000 synthetic chemicals [that] include plastics, cosmetic chemicals, pesticides, antibiotics, industrial chemicals, and other drugs… have firmly gone beyond a planetary limit into a so-called 'unsafe space.'" *The Science Times* January 20, 2022

"The parallels between second-hand smoke and synthetic fragrance use are many." Christy De Vader "Fragrance in the workplace: what managers need to know" *Journal of Management and Marketing Research*, 2009

The Situation

LIVING THIS MIRACLE EXISTENCE ON EARTH is no longer amazing. It is a fight, a fight to breathe, against an invisible enemy, one we will never be able to see. But in no way does it mean this enemy is not there. Our body tells us a different story. Some will be surprised to learn that millions of bodies tell the same story. There are articles and research that tell us a disturbing story. Our United States Declaration of Independence promises us an unalienable right to Life, Liberty and the Pursuit of Happiness. Unalienable, that which cannot be taken away. What does that truly mean, "cannot be taken away?" Who determines if it is taken away? What are they referring to when they say, "can't be taken away?" Who exactly in our government is supposed to protect this promise? Is it federal, state, or local government? Is the power in that promise and those words equal for everyone everywhere? With so many cities dotting the map of the United Sates, does each have the final vote if it is taken away? Or is it much more complicated than that?

Central to this book is the air we breathe that is scented by fragranced products that are made mostly with untested chemicals. It is about the strength of these fragrances that overtake our sense of smell and destroy our sense of taste. It is about how these fragrances and those chemicals make us feel.

In the science chapter of this book are provided many links from studies done that will reveal the chemicals included in the fragranced products used today. Some of those chemicals are on the front cover of this book. The links will provide easy to understand graphs, cite source material, and provide invaluable data from many studies to allow an educated assessment about two questions: Are fragrances dangerous? and do they bother others? We are confident our readers will have many other "why" questions after reviewing all the provided links and read what we and others are saying, have said, and continue to say.

Our ability to enjoy life with each breath we take has been taken away, poisoned, if we look at the research on chemicals used in the products we breathe. If each breath is filled with chemicals that are debated and questioned, how is our pursuit of happiness impacted? If our Declaration of Independence affords us a life of sickness that is caused by the very society that ignores it, we don't think it is such a great promise. Because of brilliant chemical engineers and scientists, there are as many invisible dangers in life as there are visible, perhaps more so. It is hard to fight what you can't see and that which occupies the air we need to breathe to sustain life. Air pollution is visible and carbon in the air can be measured, but still the fights against those agents have been long, costly, ongoing, and unresolved political battles. Many factors, including corruption, denial, ego, blindness, and the will to profit prevent progress toward a cleaner environment. Many in our governments throughout the world still debate whether air pollution or global warming even exist to the degree that we need to worry about them. It is sickening to watch our world being destroyed and governments doing little to nothing. With polluted air, all life is at risk of dying. Dying comes slowly for some, quickly for others.

Over Time

It took five billion years to create this earth as it looks today. Yet in only a brief moment in time we could destroy most, if not all, life, human, plant, and animal on land and in water. We have nuclear power plants on landscapes throughout this world. <u>Nuclear Power in the World Today</u>. A missile attack could destroy many of those in a matter of minutes and unleash a plague. A biological war could erase all mankind. What quantity of toxic chemicals is needed to poison the glaciers, lakes, reservoirs, rivers, streams, ponds, wetlands, and groundwater that would impact the world's source of life? This potential water destruction is a day in unwritten history that we fear the most. Five billion years to create. Five minutes to start a cascade of unstoppable destruction. We have such immense knowledge and power; it rivals these five billion years of history. In the movie *Lincoln* by Steven Spielberg, in one scene Lincoln, played by Daniel Day Lewis, says that he is "clothed in IMMENSE power! you will procure me those votes." Today, the governments throughout the world are clothed in immense power. These governments determine the quality of air we breathe with laws that allow and restrict dangerous substances. Even in Roman times the use of lead was known to cause sickness. And in each time since, the chemicals used to make products like fragrances have greatly impacted the health of those involved in the production, those that use the products and all the people who come into contact with those products who need the surrounding air to breathe. Those producers of products that pollute our air and water collaborate in government secrecy and deception, with corporate lawyers dancing around the issues in a way that would impress Fred Astaire. But with the advancement of technology and new and more toxic and lethal chemicals, the immense power continues to have a direct impact on each breath that individual citizens take. The use of untested chemicals in our products has spun out of control and continues to do so at a brisk pace.

Look at the garages of our neighbors. When they moved in they were spotless. Fast forward ten, twenty, maybe thirty years, and they are a garbage dump for everything that has gone through their life. Those garages are a simple example of how, without a specific clean-up plan, the build-up of stuff can become overwhelming. Overwhelming is a word we like to use to describe the air problem we have because of the size and scope of the problem, because of how long it has been avoided, ignored and forgotten. Those in government that are directly responsible for these chemicals in the products and fragrances consumers use have failed us miserably.

Out of Control

There is a stretch of the Mississippi River in Louisiana that is called "<u>Cancer Alley</u>" because of all the sickness that has been tied to it. It is a crime against human life so horrendous, that it makes one question the government's commitment to sustain our life. Maybe better said, since "Cancer Alley" only exists because governments have allowed it to, it suggests that the government is not committed to protecting and sustaining our life. We see political power bought and sold like cattle since money influences all who dare desire it. We must take back this immense power, and restore the air we breathe to what it was before industry and technology dictated that we breathe toxic air.

Our Bodies

Don't be fooled by appearances. A person who has breast cancer, leukemia, prostate cancer, muscular dystrophy, multiple chemical sensitivity, or so many other life-threatening and debilitating illnesses might look completely healthy. We say this because we never want to dismiss or question someone who says they don't feel well. Most of us aren't doctors. And still, doctors today have a lot to learn.

Our body's heart pumps approximately 2,000 gallons of blood daily. How The Heart Works. It is not something you control. You can't say, "Heart, stop pumping for a while, and take a break and rest up, extend your useful life, because I want to live until I'm a hundred and fifty years old." The normal menstrual cycle for women on average is twenty-eight days, but might be as short or long as twenty-one to forty days. This is not something an individual woman can choose. You can't say, "Menstrual cycle, stop for 30 years and then continue into my 70s or 80s because I want children much later in life." Ha ha… Menstrual cycle: What's normal, what's not. Some people are born with allergies while others develop them later in life. It is our immune system's response to a foreign substance. You can't tell your immune system, "Don't be bothered by that substance." You can't ask your immune system, "Why don't you just ignore that substance, and eventually you will get used to it." Unfortunately, most of the time, we have no say over how our immune system responds to substances. It is very important to understand that our bodies are complex and we cannot dictate many things that go on within our bodies, no matter the foods we eat or the amount of exercise we do. 12 Systems of the Body . We are complex organisms with over twelve separate systems including the skeletal, nervous, and immune systems. So, when a person says their health is affected by an odor or chemical in the air, they are chemically sensitive, it is just part of the body's system at work. Again, it's not like we can say, "Ha, immune system, stop that, you are bothering me." It is an involuntary reaction. This sensitivity can come from a single exposure, or a cumulative effect of repeated exposures as we grow older in this fragrance-chemical warfare and toxic air we breathe and battle. It grows in severity as it relates to a specific fragrance and/or chemical and it can manifest as a response to many other fragrances and chemicals. But when it happens it is our body's system warning us something is wrong. The fragrances sold today, in mass quantities, the degree of strength, the number of chemicals used to make them, including the fragrances and chemicals used to make cleaning products, have overtaken the air we breathe. They are everywhere, and seem to poison every breath we take.

Odors are and have always been a subjective sensation. Always remember that, when someone says something bothers them though it doesn't bother you.

Olfactory Fatigue

For the millions that have asked friends, family, and co-workers for fragrance consideration and have heard the answers, "I don't smell anything," or "I only put on a little," maybe the answer is in the words "olfactory numbness, olfactory fatigue, olfactory adaptation or nose blindness." These terms describe when a body becomes desensitized to stimuli, in this case, frequently used fragrances, and it prevents the person from noticing them. The two very important links "olfactory fatigue" and "the sense of smell" may be two of the most important links that we share because they will help those fragrance wearers and fragranced laundry product users to understand just how strong and offensive they do smell to someone who is sensitive to fragrances. These links are point on in their message that if a pig farmer, zookeeper, sanitation worker or roofer no longer notices the smell associated with their job, you can understand how olfactory numbness will block out all fragrance awareness from fragrance users.

The Sense of Smell

Because of the complexity of the human race, and the ever-evolving knowledge of science, Hyperosmia, an increased olfactory acuity, can never be ruled out for those who are affected by fragrances the most. We've learned a great deal about the human body these last 100 years and continue to learn at a brisk pace. But many questions still remain. Regardless of where a person falls on the scale of olfactory acuity, if a fragrance makes them uncomfortable or sick, that is what it does.

All healthy breathable air seems to have ceased to exist.

We're here to try and clean up the air we breathe and take control of our health. Let's try to remove olfactory overdoses from this overly fragranced world.

It's easy to say "it's safe," until time proves it isn't.

It is just as easy after so many have suffered and died to say, "We're sorry, we didn't know, oops, how could we not have seen that, our mistake," or the often used, get-out-of-jail-free card answers, "We will try to do better, we must do better."

You can't erase history, no matter who or how powerful you are!

It's a brisk beautiful morning. Yesterday's shopping spree of fresh ground coffee beans promises us a cup of coffee for the senses. Those coffee beans produce one of life's great joys. The taste, exceptional, but the smell, wow, doesn't do it justice. Time for a walk. We are barely out the front door and someone is walking toward us from the opposite direction. Bam, punched with an odorant that punishes our senses. Our olfactory sensory neurons just hit overload. Our brain goes into panic mode. We can feel our blood pressure rise. What just happened? Why do we suddenly feel sick? Minutes go by and slowly we feel our normal self coming back. Conscious, we know we were punched. Sadly, we feel like boxers, but boxers whose lives are constantly lived in the ring. And our sparring partners live around every corner, and are constantly throwing punches that connect dead center on our nose. Our brain is always rattled in confusion. This book will explain why it is we, the fragrance-chemical-sensitive, feel the way we do, and hopefully shed light on how life outside the ring could and should be possible.

Or maybe it's been done already and proven to work? On September 26, 1991, and ending September 26, 1993, a team of eight started a two-year experiment living inside Biosphere 2.

Comments from Jane Poynter, who helped design and then lived in this 3-acre dome called Biosphere 2, upon exiting the controlled environment:

"I run over to say hello to all of these people and reel back," Jane Poynter said in an interview with Bizwomen. "We all stink from all the chemicals we put on our bodies. It wasn't that we didn't have shampoo or toothpaste [in Biosphere 2], but it was all very organic, no perfume, no hairspray."

Biosphere 2

That comment, "we all stink," why didn't those three telling, powerful words get anyone's attention? Was anyone in government listening? When we watch the news today, we hear the same stories months on end. Why aren't the news producers doing a better job of showing a real time picture of life on earth instead of a repeated picture hundreds of times? The four o'clock hour announcer said the exact same things as the five o'clock hour and the six o'clock hour does it again. In our opinion, those words, "we all stink," is news worth telling. News outlets should breathe in fresh new content on the condition of our air until we all can breathe clean air. Who in the news business has the courage to tell in real time today's story of what we breathe?

If we go back to Biosphere 2 we ask ourselves, why didn't they put fragrances and the chemicals used to make our daily products in Biosphere 2? Why did they conduct a very costly and important experiment excluding the true air conditions of Biosphere 1, Earth? Why did they conduct an experiment impossible to duplicate here on earth?

Why do we all stink? And what does our air smell like?

Does the cigarette industry come to mind when you think about the air we breathe or used to breathe? Raise your hand if you'd like to go back to the days of smoke-filled cars, trains, airplanes, homes, and workplaces. Before the enlightenment about the dangers of tobacco, every workmate, classmate, and family member had a cigarette between their fingers filling up the environment with smoke. The smell of cigarettes was pervasive on people, on clothes, in public places. Thankfully, that has changed in many places. Sadly, smoke has been replaced with the overuse and abundance of fragranced products cloaking and choking us, as did smoke.

The Paradigm of Sharing Fragrances

EVERY SECOND OF EVERYDAY A SORT of crime is committed. Yet, as far as history shows, no one has been arrested, jailed, or taken to court for it. At least, we have not read about it on the front-page news, or the back page news. It's not news. But the way that people wear fragrances with abandon and sicken others should be a crime.

We think the most important two questions that need to be answered if we, as a society, are going to see the value in this book are: Does the scent coming off you affect others in a negative way? Is your personal scent, a chemically powerful combination of personal care products, harmful for you to use and harmful for those around you?

How does one protect oneself so they don't come home smelling like ten other people? We should rephrase that question; How does a person protect themself so they don't come home smelling like what we will learn is "Intrusive Potion #12, 15, 20, etc.?"[1] A baseball pitcher with a good combination of three or four pitches is one who puts fear in hitters. Should we fear the combination of fragrances and chemicals coming off of the people with whom we intersect?

So, is it possible to protect yourself from these fragrances and hundreds or possibly thousands of chemicals, should you not want to smell like "Intrusive Potion #15"?

To understand and visualize what a person smells like, we like to imagine taking a large bowl, and pouring in and mixing all the fragranced products most people start their day with. These are the products that people put directly on their skin or use to scent their clothing. Examples of these products include shampoo, conditioner, straightener, face soap, body soap, deodorant, lotions, perfume, cologne, shaving cream, hair spray, makeup, laundry products (labeled "triple-strength"), fabric softeners, dryer sheets (labeled "long-lasting"), bleach, stain remover, and "odor eliminator" with scent booster, etc., etc. What is the final count on the fragranced products you use? Is it ten, fifteen, or twenty-one products that emit a scent? This intrusive potion in a fragrance wearer's bowl is their signature scent. This scent is what announces them to the world. Does anyone really know what their signature smell is? It's funny but also

---

[1] We refer to the "intrusive potion" with random numbers to indicate that each person uses a multitude of mingling scents each day (also known as "the punch bowl" or "the chemical soup") which becomes a mixture they probably did not intend but has very negative effects on those around them.

very sad to think what a triple-strength laundry detergent and someone's expensive and cherished perfume smell like when combined. If scents were neon, they would blind most.

We wonder should it be a crime to be a second-hand fragrance spreader and air polluter of chemicals that make up their intrusive signature scent that they apply to start the day? Is it not true that second-hand smoke is a crime in most areas now? Though we wonder how many tickets are given out annually across the United States to those who break the law on smoking in public. We ask this question because it has been many years since smoking in public has been banned in most areas. And if laws and rules are not enforced, what value do they serve? We will explore this later in the book when we talk about fragrance-free policies. But for now, let's get back to the paradigm of sharing fragrances and its impact on others.

We call the "chemical-fragrance criminal" the "Hug Attacker" and "Spreader."

When fragrance wearers leave their house, they decide they want to smell heavily fragranced. Even one spray of those potent perfumes or colognes that last all day will surely announce their presence. Triple-strength laundry detergents let people know they are coming hundreds of feet away. But isn't that the purpose of what they are doing when they fragrance up, to be smelled? Fragrance wearers fragrance themselves so others will smell them for as long as we are in their presence. We think it's safe to say that they don't use fragrance just for themselves. Who lounges around the house in PJs to read the paper on Sunday morning with the same Monday morning ritual of cosmetics and perfumes? The morning ritual should put a 100% stamp of certainty on the realization that they, the fragrance wearers, understand the reason they use fragrances. They use fragrances to announce their presence with a long-lasting invisible cloud of chemical scent, one that will last long after they have gone, and announces them long before they arrive. What was the formula they used? "Intrusive Potion #14" or was that "Intrusive Potion #21"? The combination of fragranced products will include hundreds if not thousands of potentially untested chemicals. In conclusion, if you are a fragrance user, you are a second-hand fragrance spreader.

The "Hug Attacker"

What category of attacker are you? A "serial" hugger? A "sneak up behind hugger?" A "must say hello to everyone" hugger like at the Academy Awards? We can see that there are so many choices, so many chemicals, and so many intrusive potion mixes.

Another important question the fragrance wearers must ask themselves, do others want to smell like them, the fragrance wearer? They must be aware that since they did put on those fragrances to smell how they like to smell, that others they hug will then have that same "Intrusive Potion# 15" on them. Now as the day goes on, one "Hug Attack" at a time, the more of a "Hug Attacker" one is, the more their signature scent changes. And the more they collect, the more the fragrance grows in strength and chemical impact. It's easy to smell intrusive Potion #16 turning into Intrusive Potion #100 after just a few rounds of Hug Attacking. So, whether one attacked or was attacked, both yield the same result: fragrances were shared, mingled, and created new potentially strong fragrances.

Generally, men and women choose different types of fragrances, but all is for nought once they hug or touch someone else. There is no longer a masculine smell and a feminine smell, but some kind of combination smell. Each "Hug Attack" with that double arm embrace for ten seconds rubs their signature scent and chemical load onto the other. As a young boy I remember the anxiety of having to hug Grandma and Grandpa with their off the charts signature smells. Has anyone else had that same anxiety?

Let's count how many places fragrances can be exchanged from one person to the next or have lasting power long after that person is gone.

1. Handshaking is an easy example to visualize this sharing of fragrances. Though we should replace the word: "hand-shake" with "fragrance-chemical shake."

2. Being hug-attacked is where maximum fragrance exchange occurs.

3. We pick up a great deal of a person's fragrances just standing next to them.

4. When one sits down, they sit where others also sat and left an attacking part of their signature scent. This sitting includes going almost anywhere that isn't one's own private furniture. A few places that come to mind include a doctor's office, shopping areas, salons, and restaurants. Forty minutes in the dentist chair after "Intrusive Potion #21" just left, and we both say we would take root canal without novocaine over that chair.

5. How about getting packages that the delivery services leave on the doorstep? Those packages, touched and carried by several individuals, arrive cloaked in fragrances. The hallway fills with a sillage[2] that clings, lasts, and waits to attach itself to any innocent victim.

6. Try signing for packages with a pen that carries the scent of the worker and all their previous clients. It is amazing just how much of an attaching scent comes off a pen as one panics and worries about how they are going to immediately get that smell off their hand.

7. Standing in line with people is also standing in line with fragrance sillages, which, doing their job, cling to others.

8. When people carry luggage or handle the things an individual will touch or take home is another open avenue for fragrance sharing. Hands, as we will learn in another section, are an enemy that leaves fragrance mines on everything it touches. Like the pen, touch it, and an explosion of fragrances grips the hand, and one may wish to blow it off like a landmine.

9. The fragranced sales clerk who handles clothes at check-out is a fragrance spreader. Why does the sales person always use their chest to help fold the clothes? The chest is a breeding ground for fragrances that find a new home on new clothes.

10. Riding in people's cars or taking other forms of transportation is the perfect storm for a fragrance spreader. Parking valets seem to be some of the worst fragrance offenders. Do they think the stronger the scent, the bigger the tip? Then there are the people who need to get in one's car for needed repairs, oil changes, car washing, or tune-ups. Every person who drives and/or enters the car, exits at some point, and leaves their signature sillage, plus the scents from their clothes

---

[2] Sillage is the trail or the wake of a perfume left behind in the air of the wearer

on anything they touch or sit on. A pair of pants cleaned in laundry detergent with the most offensive smelling fabric softener added, will mean a day's worth or a week's worth of smelling someone else's clinging fragrance landmine on the car seats. Somehow one needs to clean out that intrusive scent from those seats (impossible to do as the valet pulls up your car), every pair of pants you wear, as they explode with that intrusive laundry scent as soon as contact is made. And the nightmare repeated scenario to remove it will begin.

11. We often wonder how athletes handle other smells before important sports events when they are required to shake hands with officials and many others? Basketball players shake hands with celebrities in the front row seats, or football players in the center of the field shake hands with opposing players and the referees. There are many occasions in special sporting events where the field of potential handshakes and the "intrusive hug" come very much into play. Do these encounters impact performance? We've seen athletic performances by great athletes that never made sense to us. We ask ourselves, was their performance impacted by the fragrances from handshakes and hugs with others?

12. Occasions like award shows where "Hug Attacking" is done before someone performs, or after someone accepts an award, are fertile ground for fragrance sharing. Are musicians affected by the transferred substances to their hands? How does an Academy Award winner give an acceptance speech when they are attacked by the fragrances from the hug attack as they are presented their award? We've seen many horrible acceptance speeches. Did those fragrances have something to do with it? We both love classical guitar and Ana Vidovic is an all-time favorite of ours. Her intensity and concentration appear to be beyond human. Her hands express every breath she takes. What would be the performance impact should her hands smell of someone's strong fragrance? Does the everyday "Hug Attacker" transferring the fragrances onto others affect people's daily performance or mood? Does it impact the way they treat others? Some people just seem moody at the drop of a hat. Are attacking fragrances making them moody, without the realization that they are sensitive to fragrances, without putting two and two together? It shouldn't come as a surprise to many, or maybe it should, but anyone just might be sensitive to fragrances because of how they make one feel.

So, we ask an important question, do "Hug Attacks" bother people, performers, athletes, and people in everyday life, both consciously or unconsciously?

Signs of chemical sensitivity include disorientation, confusion, hyperactivity, headaches, increased irritability, chest pains, breathing problems, loss of balance, and more. For us it is hard to see how these fragrance spreader events don't play a major role in the daily lives of people, professional or not. It might be surprising to learn in the attached studies that they definitely do. And when we add those who don't understand yet why it is they feel awful, the number of people negatively affected by fragrances grows much larger.

13. Outside the door to our house are packages of products bought online. But each package comes with a problem: it is scented by everyone who has touched it, including smokers. Too often we see our delivery company's employees smoking in delivery trucks on their daily routes. Our entire front door area fills with this scent as it looks for all possible openings to announce itself in our

home. As we sit eating a meal or watching TV, much too often we ask, where is that smell coming from? Only to realize in our search to remove it or shut every window, that it is a package left on our doorstep, as we didn't hear it being delivered.

14. What are the perils of taking in clothes to the tailor or the dry cleaner? Do they come back drenched in the tailor's scents and their table's scents from all the piles of mingled clothes worked on? You bet they do!

Many people live in the public's eye and it is often the case that touching, shaking hands, hugging, kissing, sitting with and traveling together are everyday affairs. This involuntary sharing of fragrances brings a chemical war to the everyday worker. Consider those coffee shop business meetings where colleagues sit on couches and chairs that hundreds just this past week sat in with the fragrances they leave behind. Of course, also consider the groomed or ungroomed dogs that inconsiderate owners allow to sit on the furniture too. Who wants to smell like a dog?

If someone is sprayed by a skunk, the antidote is to bathe in tomato juice. Not everyone has met a roofer, but all know the strong smell of tar. There is no antidote. It is a smell roofers live with. Is anyone ready to get "Hug Attacked" by a roofer and be okay with how they smell? Each person's "signature scent" could make people sick and feel uncomfortable, the same as a non-roofer would feel, walking around smelling like a roofer. If a person needs to live fragrance- and chemical-free, how do they remove those smells from their everyday life?

In the war of fragrance sharing, how much is a person's health impacted, both short- and long-term, by constantly being hug-attacked? Do they lose days or weeks or months or years? We only have to look at 9/11 or information from the Gulf War and its Burn Pits to understand that the health impact from these severe situations come at differing times and severity per person. But there is strong evidence that chemical exposure comes with devastating consequences. Comparing the devastating health consequences of a 9/11 first responder with those of people negatively affected by everyday fragrances may seem extreme, but we find it helpful to put ourselves in someone else's shoes. We both find clarity in life when we imagine walking in someone else's shoes.

We have mentioned the seemingly unlimited fragranced products being used by people, from scented soaps and perfumes to hair products and laundry detergent. From experience we've all learned how long some of these smells can last. The intrusiveness on the senses is unrelenting, powerful, over the top, nonstop, to the point that nothing can seem to remove this sensory overload and what it does to people after being exposed to it.

The Money Factor

Money certainly is a major component to spreading fragrances. The journey of a dollar bill and its story might reach Hollywood someday if that journey reaches the pen of a gifted writer. How many fragrances, good or bad, depending on the reader's opinion of what good or bad is, touch a dollar bill? Let's follow the journey of a dollar bill used by a gardener who spreads manure and/or chemical fertilizers and pesticides with their hands. We have all read many articles on the health risks associated with these chemicals. Since we are talking about their hands, we might as well think back to their early morning ritual and what products they may put on their hands before the work day starts: cologne, fragranced lotion, soap, and aftershave. They probably fill up the lawnmower, weed cutter and other machines with gas, another odorous product their hands touch throughout the day. This is their signature smell. Lunchtime comes and the gardener heads to the nearest food truck, pulls out their wallet and with these very used hands pulls out the money needed to pay for lunch. These dollar bills land into the hands of the food truck person who normally does it all. Their day might begin with cleaning the truck with special chemicals. Some might use gloves, but many do not. To them, those chemical smells are just part of their day. And yes, their early morning routine started the same as the gardener's, or just about everyone on the planet. The gardener's dollar bills are exchanged for food and perhaps some change in the form of dollar bills from the food truck vendor. Each dollar bill exchanged for food or other items carries a chemical load.

Other people who handle money are roofers, fragrance counter salespeople, factory workers, industrial waste haulers, etc., etc. In other words, we can begin to understand that the exchange of paper money in these hands over and over and over again is a spreader of fragrances beyond the scope of comprehension. We do not use cash. It literally sickens us.

Furthermore, does anyone regularly wash their wallet? Those designer leather women's bill holders that cost thousands of dollars and in turn probably carry lots of cash, do they ever get cleaned? Can those expensive leather bill holders even be cleaned without ruining the leather? Inside, the satin-covered bill compartment, that sees a constant exchange of bills over many years, must have a powerful scent to it. It probably amounts to thousands of chemicals that have come into contact with those dollar bills.

We often observe a cash register, a bank money bag, a mail carrier bag. We've been in thousands of stores in our lifetime, and have seen many armored security trucks pick up and deliver money. Yet, we don't recall ever seeing a cash register or money bag that looked like it has been cleaned or dusted on a regular basis. Just walk into any post office or delivery service company, and look at the bags that hold packages, packages which in turn have been touched by the many human hands we've been talking about. Do they look like they are cleaned regularly, or ever?

We are living through COVID as we write this book. It seems nothing stops the spread of the virus. How much did money play a part in its spread?

The Auto Transfer

How many people's fragrances are involved in the delivery of a new car? We can start at the manufacturing facility, and move down the line as follows to the shipping port, truck delivery to car dealer, service, test drives, final cleaning, and the delivery to the showroom of car dealer for pickup. With people and cleaning products, how many fragrances has the new car been introduced to, not to even mention the chemical coating on all the new materials? The very last delivery comes from an excited sales person trying to look and smell their best so that clients remember them. So, as a gift, the new car will have their special

"Intrusive potion #19" to drive home with. Personally, we were shocked to find out that our brand-new RV was driven 2,000 miles from the plant to the dealer by an individual driver who spent days and days leaving his chemically-fragranced footprint throughout our new "home."

A friend told us a story about how he bought his uncle's old car. As he laughed, we knew and he knew that it was more out of horror than joy. After two years with more cleanings than he could count, he could not get his uncle's signature "Intrusive Potion + cigars" smell out of the car. He was haunted by his uncle and his scent.

The Joy of Getting Presents

Who doesn't like to get a present? It brings joy and surprise and a warm heart knowing someone cares. But how do we receive presents that are drenched in others' fragrances? It is impossible to bring into our home even the smallest of presents if it smells like "Intrusive Potion #19." We wonder "where did they keep it that it smells so strong?" Perhaps while traveling some like to buy presents and put them in the suitcase that is filled with laundry-product-drenched clothes and bottles. Some buy them and store them in the clothes closet until the time is right to share the joy of giving. Very unfortunately, they are giving much more than the present. Presents today, from a simple cooked dinner in a storage container that has been cleaned in fragranced dish soap to a box of chocolates placed on the car seat with the overpowering "Intrusive Potion #17" smell of that person filling the inside car air, to their handling the box makes it impossible to accept any present. Trying to explain this to people that we care about is like pulling teeth from a hungry lion. But we just don't want to feel sick or live in the spotlight of their fragrances.

Bow Please

Do we need a hello and goodbye cultural change? COVID has taught us that human contact is a germ spreader. We know that handshakes and hugs are fragrance spreaders. What is wrong with a simple bow to say hello and goodbye with hands clasped together? One can say "namaste" or "greetings to you," or bow with any phrase from "hi," "bonjour," "buenos días," or any language you speak. The bow shows respect.

In other words, we wish that others would please keep their fragrances, made from mostly untested chemicals, to themselves, as well as their germs and viruses. Because of COVID, people are starting to understand that their hug could be the cause of someone else's getting sick even though it was out of kindness. When one is chemically sensitive, one really appreciates social distancing. If we were to switch to the nonphysical bow, we might see a dramatic decrease in people catching the flu, a cold, or the dreaded fragrance transfer.

Please Sit

We, as a couple, no longer go to movie theaters, plays, concerts, or any indoor arena. Who might be sitting next to us, in front of us, behind us, with too much horrifying fragrance? Who sat in the same seat for three hours before we did and before that? It is unimaginable to spend three hours in close contact with fragranced people in almost any setting.

The joy we get from riding our trikes is unmatched. Four years ago, we decided to put motors on them because Biker Bob lives with Muscular Dystrophy and its degenerative progression. We always wish we could share our experiences with others. We used to have two extra trikes for this very reason. But the reality of letting someone sit on our trike seats with fragranced clothes and hold onto the grips with fragranced hands always stopped us from sharing our love of our favorite activity. We want to share our love but we do not want to share fragrances.

Being Your Best

Most everyone around us is filling our senses with fragrance-chemical overload. Sometimes we may ask ourselves, "Why wasn't I at my best today? I felt good as I left the house." For many, putting on fragrances is a habit that they perform without consciousness. Aristotle said it best, "We are what we repeatedly do. Excellence, then, is not an act, but a habit." Applying "Intrusive Potion #17" might very much contribute to how a person feels, but it is ignored as a factor. Someone might think, "Why are my allergies so bad? I always feel a little stuffed up. It must be the foods I'm eating, that has to be why my chest hurts." My wife embarrassingly admits that she used to put perfume on the back of her neck so that it wouldn't bother her. Now, we both have the same reaction every time we are out walking, riding, or driving with the windows down and our air space is invaded by a passerby's perfume or cologne, "pu!"

Shopping

THE COMPETITIVE NATURE OF SELLING PRODUCTS makes each retail store an opportunity to attract people, and these days, a signature scent for places seems to be a retail must. Not only does the space in general need to have a smell, but also we see the most potent smelling devices that plug into every free outlet, especially in the restroom. Some of the large retail stores have huge fragrance and cosmetic departments. Those fragrances and thousands of chemicals create an invisible cloud overtaking the air and therefore, a fragrance and chemical foundation that coats the entire store's contents. One walks through these departments and witnesses people spraying perfumes and aftershave to see if they like the smell. No concern is given to the millions who are sensitive and aware of the harmful effects of fragranced products. Should the blame go to the stores that still allow this spraying and testing ritual? Bringing home any item from these stores is much more than we bargained for, and in our house, it sets off a ritual to decontaminate it. Other smaller retail stores sell only their signature fragrance brand. Some of those brands' fragrances are so powerful, so potent, so intrusive, and so unmistakable (which we guess is their intent), that even in outdoor shopping areas, these fragrances can be detected from hundreds of feet away in all directions. Inside shopping malls, those smells reach every level above and below, left to right as this intrusive smell leaves its chemical-fragrance mark. Each walk by is a chemical-clinging assault that is impossible to avoid. What law gives them the right to fill the air up with such a heavily fragranced chemical-induced smell that it is unavoidable? It's like walking into a group of smokers, without a choice. Who today wants to be subject to those chemicals and, most importantly, have no choice? If someone should suffer a massive headache from those fragrances and chemicals, do the stores have responsibility? Should they have a responsibility to the public for this fragrance-chemical cloud?

The smell of new clothes depends again on where you buy them. As mentioned, some stores have a smell that is unmistakable. This must stem from the variety of products they carry, and where these products are placed in the store and where they were made. Others sell those fragrances that seem to embed into the clothing so that when we take them home, those fragrances are again unmistakable and identifiable to that retailer. But even before the clothes reach the retailer to add those additional fragrances to the clothing, clothing manufacturers use a variety of chemicals in the manufacturing process, including formaldehyde. New rain gear, synthetic clothing, and the smell of new panniers are smells that are hard to miss. The off-gassing of chemicals from these products is overwhelming. New shoes produce a chemical cloud so strong, that if they were running shoes, their smell would come in first for a race to the senses. In our experience, we have brought home two new pairs of running shoes and the off-gassing of one pair is off the charts offensive, while the other is barely noticeable. A big why? Where is the information we need to protect ourselves? We have the right to know what these chemicals are and how much of them is being used in our products. Are manufacturers using chemicals that alarmingly harm the health of their workers and their consumers?

Considered Chemistry at Nike

We are so proud of the Green Chemistry and Commerce Council for the transparency they used in the above linked case study entitled "Considered Chemistry at Nike: Creating Safer Products through the Evaluation and Restriction of Hazardous Chemicals." Nike, in its effort to become a more sustainable brand, has also become a brand that seeks to "find better ways to evaluate materials and produce products that are safer for consumers and the environment."

Other shoe makers recently have said they are removing some chemicals from the manufacturing process. Others haven't said "boo." The off-gassing that we have to contend with, with almost every shoe we've ever bought, spells "boo!" to us because the chemical load reaches deep inside our throats and lungs and irritates them for hours. Exactly what chemicals are they removing and why? Is it because of the harm those chemicals caused in all those years of our buying those shoes? Why did it take so long? Why did our government stand by and watch, and allow chemicals with "harmful potential" and "unanswered questions about [their] toxicity to humans" to go on for so long? What did the studies show about the toxicity of those chemicals to the workers and the wearers? Have studies been done on the likelihood of cancer to those workers as compared to workers in the same areas but in different industries that aren't subject to working with and breathing in those chemicals in question? When we look at Ground Zero from 9/11, all those present were greatly affected by the chemicals in the air. How many excuses and "we didn't knows" have we heard from those who said "it was safe" to be around? So again, I ask for workers in factories spread across the globe, making shoes, clothes, or any product where chemicals are a big part of the manufacturing process, what is the likelihood of cancer? What cancers have been found? Have studies been done? We know that Jon Stewart had to defend the 9/11 first responders before Congress, because their health care plans were not robust enough to aid them in all the sickness they suffered as a result of exposure.

Shopping adventures are perilous when it comes to immediate health risks of those acutely sensitive. Symptoms include but are not limited to light-headedness, shrunken throat and airways, chest as tight as a new drum. These are just a few of the many signs that those chemicals have found their way to us. Besides the stores' smell on new clothes, is the horrible change in smell of the clothing you were wearing when you get home. We are amazed, shocked, and desperate when we walk in the door, and realize that the clean clothes we left the house with now smell like a fragrance overload, like "Intrusive potion #17 or #36 or worse." We don't sit down in public because that would be like sharing a space with a family of fragrance-wearing people whose scents will surely stick to our clothes like glue. This is something we've talked about in these pages before. Of course, we were not "hug attacked" because we are hug attacker avoidance experts. So, by simply walking through these stores, we are drenched in fragrances and chemicals that we did not ask for. As fragrance-free lifers, we race to get the clothes off fast and start a load in the washer with our fragrance-free laundry detergent. Being home in our fragrance-free and chemical-free environment makes fragrances spring to life in our oxygen-rich home. But getting those fragrances out of our clothes when our laundry products are fragrance-free is no easy task.

It is nearly impossible to test out furniture and survive being fragrance-free. Imagine ten people on that furniture before in the last hour; we haven't got a chance. What do we do? It isn't fair and we want to scream. It feels like our health and well-being are being unfairly attacked without anything we can do about it. We keep bringing up being attacked by others' fragrances from shared seats in a variety of situations to prove the point. It is very hard to avoid in life's daily adventures. And once fragrance-attacked, the journey for us and our clothes to return to being fragrance-free, is not an easy road to travel. It's a sad road millions travel daily.

For now, we all live in this unfair world.

Buying New Products

As mentioned above, bringing home new clothing, and all types of products, is like self-delivering chemicals inside your home. Realistically, it is almost impossible to bring home new products without a chemical-smelling overload of fragrances. Remember how smoking used to be widespread, but now people boldly guard themselves against exposure to cigarettes and second-hand smoke. For us, many conditions need to be met before a product is safe for wearing or placing in our home. We need to gauge how many washings it takes or how long it needs to hang outside before it is useable. There are actually some types of fabric that never let go of the smell. Cycling clothing and other synthetic materials are just one example.

Travel, One of Life's Delights. Or Is It?

When one is sickened by chemicals and fragrances it's not possible to risk booking an hours-long flight to a part of the world they wish they could see. Also problematic is public transportation. Not only have several fragranced people sat where they are expected to, but also, the ride-sharing drivers think that they should "smell nice" for the public. On the very last flight Bob took, because he no longer flies, the person sitting next to him spilled her perfume bottle on herself in the bathroom. For four hours he had to survive what seemed like four years. This is one of those chemical assaults that makes sensitive people fearful of life.

When we think of traveling, our worries include how bad will the fragrances be in hotel rooms, luggage compartments, and ride-share vehicles? Even stunning tourist attractions like the ruins at Machu Picchu, a boat ride up the Seine, a tour of Notre Dame can quickly become stifling and uncomfortable when people's scents take over. We are limited from enjoying even local social events like wine tasting, high school reunions, graduations, and so much more of what life offers. We are tempted to travel when we are introduced to such beautiful locations on TV, but until teleport travel is invented, we will have to settle for the virtual experience. We cannot fathom getting our luggage back permeated with fragrances. It is enough to say, "We quit, it's too difficult, we're packing it in." Or should we say, "We are unpacking this life" because of the degree of difficulty it portends. Traveling today is just not in the fragranced cards.

Comparisons Tell a Tale

We do not intend to denigrate homeless people, many of whom we believe are victims of an uncaring and capitalistic society. That is to say, when one lives in Santa Monica or is out and about in Los Angeles, one comes into contact with many, many homeless people. We know that some homeless people choose to live on the fringes of society, but there are also many others who are in dire need of help and medical care. An infirm mind does not understand the concept of personal hygiene. Their clothes and their bodies have not been washed in years. Though this is not the kind of chemically-induced smell that we have been describing, by the same token, it is a smell that would take one's breath away. It is difficult to imagine being near it for more than a moment.

It becomes harder and harder to count friends and family as part of the richness of our life. How do we fit them in our fragrance-free world? What do they smell like? Most importantly, how willing are they to change their personal hygiene habits and products to spend time with us? Most experience has shown "not much." It's not that they intend to do us harm, it is that they don't understand how a scent and the chemicals therein make us feel so bad. It seems that only a tidal wave of momentum, an awakening, could change society's habits as a whole, like what happened with cigarette smoking. If someone says that their son is allergic to peanuts, no one would dare to bring peanuts around him, or cook him something with peanuts in it. If we tell the exact same someone that we are allergic to fragrances and the chemicals in them, they are immediately offended. It's as if they didn't hear what we just said. They can't fathom that something they do not notice makes us uncomfortable and sick. But strangely, they do understand peanut allergies.

For a moment, we would like to play the Imagine Game with you, our fair reader.

Let's switch to the sense of sight. Imagine for a moment that there are bright lights shining in your eyes nonstop. You must work under these conditions, eat under these conditions, do schoolwork under these conditions, even sit on the sofa to relax under these conditions. How would this overload of light impact your performance? Your mood? Your health? No one wants a spotlight shining in their eyes all day long, especially without the ability to shut it off.

Let's examine the sense of hearing. Imagine a loud fire engine roaring down the street blasting in your ears, all day long. Imagine having this sound present as you eat, work, play, study, or read. Not one person wants a fire engine sound blasting in their ears, especially without the ability to turn it off. Both of these examples of sensory overload would be considered forms of torture.

In both of these situations, you have no say or defense in adjusting the light or sound.

You could substitute a simple flashlight or a bare light bulb for the spotlight. You could substitute a gas-powered leaf blower, a baby crying, an unending alarm clock, a teapot whistle, or a car horn for the fire engine. Even if you cut those lights or sounds in half and try to visualize yourself sitting in a restaurant eating or studying for an exam, or writing a letter, consider what your state of mind would be. We think we can all agree that such situations would amount to more than a distraction. It would be torment.

We are drawing these comparisons so that you can understand what happens when a person's sense of smell is subjected to unwanted and harmful fragrances. No one wants to smell manufactured fragrances all day long without the ability to turn their "volume" off. This sensory overload has a painfully negative effect on performance, mood, attitude, and health. Being around fragrances for us, and for millions of others, is a form of torture or abuse. We have learned that because of "olfactory fatigue," the actual offenders wearing the fragrance don't even notice it anymore. They cannot imagine the anguish they are causing all around them.

If we were to turn to the sense of taste, would you want a cloud of fragrance invading your mouth and nose every time you took a bite of your food? Because that is exactly what happens when you share the restaurant air space with fragrance wearers.

Would you believe that the CDC and many other companies have strict fragrance-free policies? Their reasons vary from concern for "the ability for workers to concentrate," "health considerations," and the intrusiveness of two key human senses, "smell and taste." Their data tells them that people "don't want to smell fragrances all day long," especially without the ability to turn them off.

Society, we will love you like family, but you need to "TURN YOURSELF OFF." We all have work to do and a life to live, and we just can't concentrate.

Going Places Has Its Risks

This is a real example from Bob's recent experience. As he enters the physical therapy room, the pain he is feeling is all-consuming. Most of the time what the therapist offers is temporary relief, a little bit of ice, an ear to bend, and exercises that will hopefully fix the problem. But on this day entering the room, the pain seems to disappear. What takes over is worse, because it is immediate, comes without warning, and can last hours, and in some cases days and weeks. We say weeks, because once fragrance-chemical-sensitive people come into contact with the chemicals in fragrances that send minds racing, every little encounter afterward is magnified. These constant changes in sensitivity can wreak havoc on marriage and all other relationships. Bob learned the carpet had just been cleaned. That physical therapy offices even have carpet, considering the allergic reaction millions get from it, is a question for many businesses today, including doctors' offices, hospital waiting rooms, etc. The fragranced compound used to clean the carpet is off the charts strong. The chemicals used are anyone's guess. When the therapist asked Bob to lie down with his face inside the hole of the massage table, all he could smell was the carpet inches from his face. Do physical therapy offices ever truly consider the patients' needs when it comes to the office environment? We truly don't think so. Besides the carpet fragrances, the therapy bed had just been wiped down with what we consider toxic-smelling wipes. A blast of bleach up the nose just for good measure. WOW! The smell is overpowering. Did Bob come to get healed, or sick?

In the news and on the internet, there are horribly alarming stories on "sick building syndrome." What are the chemicals that are making people sick? People don't get sick from clear air. It is clear that chemicals are coming from many sources. One such source is the air freshener craze. These air fresheners seem to fill every outlet in America. Even Bob's doctor's office has one in each room, and duplicates in some. Bob always comes home sicker and more frustrated than when he went. When Bob asked the doctor about it, he mentions the building manager, and deflects his need to know. Doctors, experts on question deflection.

At work one might talk with ten or maybe twenty-five people a day. In larger companies, one might also come in contact with possibly a hundred co-workers daily. It is not a substance that can be seen, but the sillage trains circle the hallways as they wrap around throats choking out most of the air. And if we dare ask for some consideration, such as, "Could you please not wear fragrances to work?" we are the ones being offensive. One cannot expect more love or consideration from co-workers than from friends and family. Even though most people sit ten feet away from co-workers, there always seems to be an "Intrusive potion #19" like a wall of fragrance that crushes the senses, unrelenting in its attack, each and every day, all day. It is like a blazing fragrance spotlight whose alarm sound is turned up, and it comes with no switches or knobs to turn it off. The lunch rooms, lobby, constantly cleaned hallway carpets, and office furniture block every turn to fresh breath freedom.

Some lines of work require much closer interaction. The film and theatre industries are two great examples in which scenes with fellow actors are intense and close. Loving embraces, kissing, dancing cheek to cheek, and sharing a close stage with a theatre company can provide for many close encounters. Unimaginable quantities of chemically fragranced makeup are applied and re-applied. Day after day, a freshly cleaned fragranced co-star comes to work ready with their "Intrusive Potion #17," to shine a bright light on some victim's senses, distract their train of thought, and wreak havoc on their balance of timing and sense of scene awareness.

Bob saw an interview with Glenn Close in which she talked about her experience as an understudy having to wear the dress of the star she was replacing. She recalled how it smelled like the star's perfume. An actress of such talent who understands at the highest level the amount of mental commitment it takes to be an actor, to be distracted by a fragrance can only distract from being their best. Bob never found out how the performance went.

We also think about taxi drivers, bus drivers, cruise ship workers, mass transit drivers, and flight attendants because these are all jobs that require one to be around a lot of different people daily. How do these workers escape the cloud of fragrances and chemicals that rise up from their passengers to reach out and grab them? Even if they aren't aware of the fragrances, they still face the potential result of sickness to follow being around all these untested chemicals.

One might think that the higher the salary, the safer the environment. But even with twenty-plus million-dollar salaries in professional sports, more money doesn't equate to safer working conditions. Basketball players bump, hold, and bounce off each other for hours during their eighty-plus games a year. American football players crush bodies as they lie in piles of human sweat tackle after tackle. In athletics, close contact is part of the game. And yet, during many interviews we've seen numerous personal care fragranced products in the lockers of athletes as they are being interviewed in the locker rooms. They come to practice and to game day with it on, and leave putting more on. Is it hard to imagine the impact these fragrances have on performance, considering what the data in the studies have shown in the links this book has provided?

We are looking for that teammate, co-star, classmate, or co-worker who challenges their cohorts to be better and healthier by saying, "Don't fragrance-cloud our focus." It could be a win-win situation.

Where are the athletes and actors of the world who have the courage to step forward for humanity's health and tell their stories on how fragrance and the chemicals impacted performance?

Where do teachers, the educators of tomorrow's leaders, run and hide as thirty high school classmates jam into a classroom trying to impress each other with "Intrusive Potion #21," a morning routine, and wrongfully perceived notion that you need to hypnotize others with scents to be attractive? School would be so much more beneficial with a "fragrance-chemical-free air" atmosphere.

Firefighters and police go to work every day not knowing if it will be their last. Firefighters have to be concerned about all the toxic chemicals swirling around inside the smoke clouds, just like 9/11. These chemicals find a comfortable resting place inside the human body. The harm they do has been documented from 9/11, to the Gulf War, to the Burn Pits that our service men and women have to tolerate. Regular people are still in the process of forcing the government to take responsibility for these illnesses. So far, the government is winning, and the service men are dying.

Millions of elderly people suffer unnecessarily due to the chemically fragranced products that their caretakers use daily. The people who need help don't get to regulate such things that would improve their air quality.

They say that our sense of smell controls mostly what we taste. But as we enter restaurants of all price points today, sitting at most tables is each person's "Intrusive Fragrance Potion." This explosion of synthetic fragrances and chemicals can and does interrupt one's enjoyment of food flavor. The next time you bite into a juicy "fragranced" burger, one of the many flavors of taste will be from that spray bottle of bright orange cleaner that untrained restaurant employees spray in mass quantities next to people's tables who are currently eating their already fragranced food. They coat the table tops with more fragrances, just to make sure when your hand touches the table, or your silverware and napkin are placed on the table, you will notice that smell on your hands. When you use the fork or the napkin you are transporting the fragrance and chemicals to your lips. Fragrances and the chemicals that make them are today's "killer of food taste."

How to Protect Oneself

There are many chance encounters, a group bike ride, standing in line, a dinner party, a daily walk, grocery shopping, where we might need to say "Stop!" before a person approaches too closely. We need to ask you some qualifying questions before we let you get close. Some of these people might be "hug attackers" whose forward progress must be obstructed. Not everyone is skilled in this screaming "stop" defense which also sometimes includes a stiff arm with tight-fisted hand. Combined, they will usually do the job in preventing fragrance transfer. Because just one "hug attack," undefended, will ensure that our brain has been taken over by a fragranced chemical alien and we will suffer for hours. But with skill and fast reflexes a person can usually stop them before they make contact. We start by explaining we are allergic to all perfumes or colognes. They might often say "I'm not wearing anything." There will probably be a change in their mood or attitude immediately. Most people just don't realize the intrusiveness of what they wear and how it affects others. They don't notice that the shampoo is made of petroleum products, or that the laundry detergent says "Triple Strength." After repeated exposure to these fragrances and chemicals, like a smoker, their sense of smell is nonexistent. They have Olfactory Fatigue and are offended that we think they smell. We must always be on our guard, ready for intrusive hug attacks with new and existing friends. We try to find new friends who understand the fragrance-free lifestyle. We look to be with people who understand the fragrance enemy, and who are living life with a sensing nose, as we wait for our governments to catch up.

An Important Distinction

Tightness in the chest and the blockage of air entering the body is a horrible feeling.

Being with others, for us, as well as for millions of sufferers, is like living with the fear that we will have to press the panic button any moment. A potential fragrance-chemical sensory attack could be around any corner, caused by someone we are with or someone they were with. It is difficult to alert friends about intrusive hugs, trying on products, or sitting in furniture without being overbearing. We sometimes unfairly get angry with our friends for not protecting us better.

We want to be crystal clear on one very important distinction. We are not saying that every exposure to fragrances causes a massive sensory overload. We are not saying that the result is always a massive headache, a constricted chest or throat, or severe confusion. What we are emphatically saying is that fragrances and the chemicals used to make them make people feel uncomfortable. They just can't seem to get them out of their mind. And this distraction does not just last a minute, but it lasts as long as they are being exposed, and afterwards if the fragrances got on them from sitting or being hugged. It can, and most often does, last long after they change clothes and shower. Using the light analogy again, a shining light that can't be avoided won't kill you, but trying to do other things while that light shines down would become challenging. That light is a distraction that makes life difficult and uncomfortable. In order to protect oneself, a fragrance-chemical-sensitive person might have to avoid many social situations that others would enjoy.

A Little Baby Story

Let's play another game. "Look in the Window"

"My name is Baby Baker, and I was just put down to nap, so Mommy and Daddy have a bedroom date. Making bedroom dates I hear is important in a good marriage. Mommy takes a shower using all her fragranced products including shampoo, conditioner, body lotion, soap, some perfume, and moisturizer. While Daddy showers using his soap, his preferred shampoo, a spray of cologne on the chest, aftershave, and some lotion for his hands, arms, and face. As they kiss, hug, and touch, all the fragrances and chemicals from Mommy and Daddy blend together. Daddy loves Mommy's breasts, so all these fragrances and chemicals embrace, mix together and rub off on Mommy's breasts. It is a magical Sunday afternoon on a rainy stay at home day. Maybe I'll have a new sister in nine months. As babies do, I start crying. "Goodbye, Daddy," Mommy says, "I love you," as she goes to get me. It's time to feed me. So, Mommy places my mouth on her fragrance-chemical-laden, horrible-tasting nipple, which I do not like. Yikes, I gasp, pull away, but Mommy insists, so back my mouth goes on that nipple. How many months must I endure this?" Sadly, this look in the window game is just everyday life. We both have personally heard stories of physicians asking nursing mothers to switch to milder soaps and detergents to stem the tide of unhappy babies and to make sure they eat. Chemicals are the opposite of the nutrition a baby desperately needs.

A Summer Breeze

Born on a summer breeze in a meadow covered in dew, first of August, I started loving you
Soon neurotoxins came your way
History's example of fragrances and chemicals at play
Lay your head down, sleep today

Born in labs, oy vey
Armies forming, tormenting
Babies cry, keep that nipple away
Tastes like fragrances and chemicals today
Nasty, an understatement, can't you hear me cry?
Stay away

Your first birthday my world turned grey
Answers, fears, a cabin's light, far away
Fragranced makeup
Shades, colors, porcelain smooth
An A.I. face
Shades of shame
Chemicals, I gave to you

A birthday wish, a candle's light
Then you left
And just like that
Dew turned to ash
And I buried you

Today's Role Models and their Message to the Young. Or are they Role Models?

The A.I., Porcelain-Smooth Colored Face

Very recently Facebook has come under fire for influencing our young in negative ways. When the people we look up to, admire, and look at as professionals feel the need to put on so much makeup as to change their identity, we need to look at who is influencing the young in the wrong direction. First on this list of those we admire are the people from the world of entertainment and television. We must also look at those who hold seats in our government's highest levels. They all are the champions of the A.I., Porcelain-Smooth Colored Face look. At concerts, the best of country music or pop sensations come on stage with that perfectly smooth as porcelain colored "A.I. Face." We've seen young senators walking through the halls of Congress being interviewed, and sometimes they are unrecognizable. They have achieved, with such expertise, that "A.I., Porcelain-Smooth Colored Face." It is a many layered application to achieve porcelain-smooth, sometimes clownishly colored, and completely different than the human face they were born with and grew up with. Invisible are all sightings of skin, freckles, blemishes, or any feature that would resemble what their morning human face would look like. Their message is so loud and so bright-colored visible, that it is no wonder why any young woman growing up through high school, college or as a professional thinks she needs to look like this too. It makes us wonder what "Intrusive Potion#?" announces to these people, considering all that fragranced, chemically-created makeup they are wearing. It must be a powerful scent. We see news anchors and senators fighting against the Facebook machine, musicians and singers, many with impressionable children of their own, stand on the world's stage signaling "see me" and "be like me." We sadly find them to be hypocrites because their faces and fragrance sillage tell a story that has a negative effect on young people and their self-image. Those in the entertainment world are so over the top with this A.I. porcelain smooth colored face because they are promoting cosmetic and fragrance companies of their own. They are the greatest influencers of this A.I. Face revolution. It means that those who are influenced must look in the mirror and decide they are ashamed of how they look. They need to imitate with fragrances and chemicals of their own.

We both wonder how today's lovers like the taste of the chemicals and fragrances applied to their partners' face and body? Is this body attractive to make love to? Do they like the chemical taste on their lips and mouth? How many people notice their lips swelling up from these chemicals? Do they like to smell like their lover after physical contact? Do lovers always like strong scents in their nose as they kiss? Are you even allowed to kiss a porcelain-smooth colored cheek today?

To use makeup says "I'm not pretty enough" or "I'm not worthy of being accepted for who I am. I need to change how I look to fit in. I won't have friends unless I look different from the face in the morning mirror. I won't be respected as a professional business person until I change how I look. My signature scent needs to be the strongest so I stand out. I need to do what everyone else does to be accepted." We strongly advocate for the clean and natural face and body. Nature's pure perfection should stand alone. Let it breathe!

What is so vitally important in this conversation is that half the world, that is billions of people, are fully accepted as nature's pure perfection. They aren't looked at as ugly. Their features aren't so hideous that they need to be covered over. Their eyes, nose, cheeks, and entire face are covered in skin. This skin also has freckles and blemishes. People don't look and feel sorry for them as they see them. They go to gala events, lavish parties, work, take their children to athletic practices, dine at fine restaurants, hike, ride bikes, and take walks. They are highly admired and respected leaders. We are talking about men. One hears he is handsome or rugged looking. People say he has a kind face. And no one comments that their skin is dried liked a prune, or looks shriveled and old before its time. To grow old is a privilege many don't reach because of illness. Men simply look like the face the mirror told them they look like first thing out of bed. Men are fully accepted in society as they are when it comes to everyday cosmetics. It is proven over a billion times a day; they just don't need them and neither do women.

Bob's Prom Challenge

Prom, is a very special day. But whose face are you going to prom with? Before you walk in the door, how many feet away should your signature scent announce you? It shouldn't. Fragrance free is the magical, invisible cloud of health, as your radiant smile announces you.

Prom is that once in a lifetime memorable day. Fill it with sharing your love. Do get a new necklace, wear the dress you made, bought, or borrowed, earrings that shine like diamonds, but aren't, a new hair style cut without chemicals or fragranced products, a signature coat and shoes to stand the test of dancing time. But most importantly, and something to be proud of for a lifetime, go with your face. Don't cover it with multiple layers of products filled with fragrances and chemicals. Be proud of who you are. Whether an athlete, musician, debater, or the most loving daughter a parent could only be proud of, you love yourself for who you are and how you look. We can always eat better, (I encourage it), exercise more, (I encourage it), try and get a few more hours of sleep, (recommended), but ultimately, you are who you are and proud of it. Freckles or none, high cheek bones, blazing green eyes or Spanish eyes that dance, you aren't trying to be anyone else. No make-up mask of chemicals is necessary because you are proud of how you look naturally. You are beautiful, you are special, you are you. Your radiant smile makes you beautiful. In spirited passionate conversation, half listening, half participating, always striving to learn from others conversation, that is where true beauty shines. Wear your face proudly with confidence like men do. Let your skin breathe, remove those unwanted chemicals that cause harm to so many and dance your way into a healthier future.

Want prom to be the most special of nights? Invite, if you can, someone who didn't plan on going to join you and your date or your group. Boy, girl, or those who identify as other, it doesn't matter. Some can't afford it, weren't asked, or just don't have the courage to go. If you can, buy them what they need or help make it, share what you already have or be resourceful and ask others for help. Spread your love to someone who needs it more than you. You will get double the joy in return, a heart filled with "I did good tonight." Look at that person, they smile, you smile. Giving is the greatest gift of all. Give the world your face to love and they will.

Prom night should be no different than all other nights and days in your life. Be that fragrance - chemical free hand, "face," "body," that reaches out and helps others. Live a life to be proud of!

I Wish I'd Known

I wish I'd known, many years ago

Goodbye my love

I wish I'd known a choice needed to be made

Goodbye my love, oh, how I love you so

They don't know, or so they say

When will we know?

They won't say

I love you so

Why do you have to go so soon?

I'll miss you so

Chemicals the reason, too many they say

Of which they don't know

Can't say, won't say

In combinations they suspect, now they say, stay away

Why couldn't you stay

Why did you have to go?

Oh Mommy, how I loved you so

School's okay, I'll make you proud

I'll try and speak out loud for those that don't

You'd be happy to hear

I went to prom last week

With my face, my beautiful face

The face the morning mirror says hello

Oh, how I loved you so

A Story Called Cigarettes

As per the American Cancer Society, tobacco smoke is made up of more than 7,000 chemicals, including over 70 known to cause cancer. Harmful Chemicals in Tobacco Products

It is not shocking news that humans have evolved from millions of years ago. One of the earliest humans is Homo Habilis or "handy man," who lived about 2.4 million to 1.4 million years ago. So, species do evolve but this evolution is not noticeable in our lifetime.

However, one thing that has changed drastically and visibly is the prevalence of cigarette smoking, at least in the United States. We can look back at pictures and see that eighty to a hundred years ago, most people smoked. We believe that 1957 was a banner year for cigarette sales. If you turn on an old movie it seems like every actor is holding a cigarette. Whether they were driving a car, working, relaxing, conversing or eating, cigarettes were a commonplace, everyday thing.

Apparently, smoke didn't bother most people when smoking was fashionable. But smoking today is considered nasty, unhealthy, and intrusive, especially in California. What happened? Knowledge. We became educated on the harm of cigarettes to the smoker and the danger of second-hand smoke to others. And it is that education that has made it so that smoking, which used to be socially acceptable, is now banned in most indoor areas and frequently such regulations are being added to outdoor areas. College campuses are non-smoking environments, as well as outdoor shopping centers and even the entire beach is smoke free. When we were growing up, both of our parents smoked around us kids without a thought. Today, ask someone if they could ride in the back seat of an enclosed car with smokers. The answer might come with some verbal abuse to even suggest it. People, you have changed.

"More doctors smoke Camels" was the cigarette brand's motto in 1947. Reading that advertising line today is extremely perturbing.

The cigarette industry dramatically demonstrated, and continues to demonstrate, the force of advertising in the United States. We have provided this information in the links below. They have tracked millions of individual purchases every day of the year and every consumer is oversold as they specify their brand by name. The rise and fall of every brand of consequence has been traced in detail and their year-to-year success or failure shown to be the direct result of consumer advertising. Today's cigarette advertising is more regulated, but it is the same loud message.

Nowadays with social media messages flooding our brains as advertising now comes in so many different avenues, we are constantly bombarded. With everything written today and understood about the dangers of smoking, that people continue to smoke is something hard to understand, unless one firmly grasps and understands just how powerful advertising is. So, it shouldn't come as a surprise that the dangers of fragrances and the chemicals that make them, and how they make people feel, isn't a topic to turn many heads yet. What does the Surgeon General say about smoking? How many deaths are attributed to smoking yearly? And with all that knowledge our governments say it's still okay to sell cigarettes. With that said, why would the government stop the fragrance and chemical industry from selling products that might cause harm? We know from the studies, the reports, and the statistics (provided below), that fragrances very much do bother people. So, waiting on our government to protect us is not logical.

People need to protect themselves by choosing more carefully what they use.

The cigarette industry used the "four dog defense" in order to continue making profits in spite of the truth being revealed about their product. It could be what the chemical industry is applying right now.

Below are two fascinating studies on the cigarette industry and how the delay game of the four dog defense works.

The Four Dog Defense

Argument one is my dog doesn't bite. When it is proved otherwise, argument two is my dog may bite but it didn't bite you. Next, my dog bit you but it didn't hurt you. And finally, OK, my dog bit you and hurt you but it wasn't my fault.

Copy of a Study of Cigarette Advertising Made By J.W. Burgard, 1953

This 60-page document gives year by year detail of just how many cigarettes were sold and how many of the population smoked. It speaks to the amount of advertising needed to reach the public, where they advertised and the cost to do so. Fascinating in its clarity, it details the advertising wars and how companies knew that it was the advertising dollars, the ads reaching the buying public, that was the key to success. It chronicles in such detail what the growth of certain brands looked like and how they influenced others to follow. It talks about how they always looked for changes like the cigarettes' size and adding a filter.

Our point is that with advertising, companies spend lots of money to flood the brains of the buying public, and they will buy. Even if it kills them. Are they doing the same with the synthetic chemicals used to make the fragranced products we wear and wash with? The advertisers say "know your buyer and you can sell them anything, harmful or not."

A study of People's Cigarette Smoking Habits and Attitudes

Cigarette second-hand smoke is understood now. That is why smoking is no longer allowed at baseball games, in restaurants, in airplanes or airports. In other words, something that used to be commonplace is now shunned.

Though there still are smokers. According to scientific studies, smokers may lose their sense of smell and taste. This might explain why a smoker tends to use double or triple the amount of fragrances. So, smokers may subject others to a high dosage of second-hand scent as well as their second-hand smoke.

Goodbye Yesterday

When we watched Peter Jackson's documentary "The Beatles: Get Back" we could almost smell the cigarette and cigar smoke that was so pervasive.

"Yesterday," when all my friends smoked the days away. Cigarette butts and ashtrays, table tops of yesterday.

cloaked in hell's cigarette and cigar smoke

Guitars that rang out yesterday

Fading, but fading not fast enough, cigarettes and cigars, be gone

you will only be that of yesterday.

Yesterday's trouble, a puff, a spray, please, go away

I declare and say, fragrances and chemicals, fade away?

You to belong to yesterday.

Let those fragrances and chemicals die on shelves today

Collect dust, no one's buying they say

Go away, you belong to yesterday

Everyone is starting to believe in tomorrow, today

Lungs breathe fresh air

People are happy

A better world, more and more say

Fragrances and chemicals

Go away, stay away

We'll live in a happier world

Fragrance-free, I think I'll stay

Take a Breath

Can't wait for tomorrow, today.

Goodbye yesterday

In this New Blue-Sky World Today

"Imagine" there's no fragrances

it's easy if you try

No sillage fragrance clouds circling us

Above a new blue sky

Imagine all the people

Smelling clean air today

You may say I'm a dreamer

But I'm not the only one

No room for fragrances and chemicals

In bathrooms of today

No spray bottles that douse

We don't splash to start the day

Come join us

In this new blue-sky world today

Living life fragrance-free

It's easy if you try

You may say I'm a dreamer

But I'm not the only one

Fragrance-Free Movement Policies

WE READ ABOUT FRAGRANCE-FREE POLICIES but have to ask, does anyone smell fragrance-free policy supervision? Fragrance-free, like smoke-free, only means something if it is enforced. Otherwise, it is 100% worthless words.

Bob's own personal experience recently at a hospital was a nightmare. First, he started screaming at a nurse while being wheeled into the operating room as her fragrances overwhelmed his senses and "scent" his brain into panic mode and his mood into attack mode. Even before that he had to use the rest room before checking in, and the moment he stepped foot into the restroom he was overcome with air freshener scent from the devices that plug into electrical sockets. They attacked him with such intensity it put an immediate horrible taste in his mouth that made him bolt for the door and give up needing to use the restroom. It is amazing how quickly our lips respond with that chemical tingling and swelling feeling. Already stressed for his upcoming spine surgery, he fought with everything inside him to keep it together. And his hospital nightmare journey ended when he left the hospital in a wheelchair pushed by a very nice man whose fragrances filled hallway after hallway. He said his heart raced, his throat started to close, his senses were on overload, but unable to walk on his own, he was forced to endure. This is due in part to a hospital ignoring the health of its patients and its so-called fragrance-free policies. Hospitals cannot claim to have fragrance-free policies if they do not enforce them. This is like a police force whose police just drive around in cars, ignoring everything they see and refusing to respond to radio requests for help. What a world that would be. It's not like the supervisors in the hospital don't know people are using fragrances. They ignore it, most likely because they use fragrances themselves. Fragrance strength today is hard to miss as it seems to grow stronger with each passing year. There is such a lack of pride in this country in doing the right thing, it pours over into every corner of society. Or with smells, it fills up every corner of every room.

How does the CDC operate under the guidelines of an extensive fragrance-free policy for all its employees and not demand the same for the world? True, they don't control the world, but they do have a gigantic platform and massive influence in society. The CDC is daily front-page news on the Covid virus. This shows that if they wanted to educate the world on this important fragrance-free policy it would not be difficult. If anything, they could highly recommend it, loudly suggest it with new laws being drafted under its supervision to protect the rest of the world's workforce. What is it that brought them to this decision to protect their workers from fragrances and chemicals? What is it they are not sharing with the rest of the world? Why would such a restrictive policy be put in place if not for the harm that fragrances and chemicals could cause its workforce? Or is the reason that how much more productive people could be working in a fragrance-chemical-free environment? The CDC at one and the same time appears to stand idle as harmful products are sold yet restricts their use by all of its employees. Are they pushing as hard as possible to eliminate those products with the lawmakers who are supposed to help protect us from harmful products? Does it appear that our laws and government agencies are protecting us?

The Science

THE MORE WE READ THE MORE WE saw the magnitude and size of the problem. The sheer number of studies on fragrances and the chemicals that make them is astounding. The places to find these studies, daunting at the start, seem to be endless. We wanted to keep reading and to keep searching but more doesn't always mean better. We have been reading medical journal after journal, from years so far back that we would think that a definitive answer to the problem would have been written by now. All of the authors seem to quote or make reference to the other researchers' studies, because the work has been done. Anne Steinemann, a civil and environmental engineering academic, is an encyclopedia of knowledge and unmatched in the volume of her studies and their results. Research is very expensive and time consuming. That is why the chemical and fragrance world continually asks for more and more research. The answers from the studies done are crystal clear. We know where the problems are. We know what needs to be done to fix the problems. We understand what it will take to save lives and to prevent suffering.

We have included a number of links below that might seem overwhelming, but we wanted our readers to be aware of our research sources. Likewise, we encourage our readers to examine the articles themselves at their own pace. Bob found that just one of Anne Steinemann's papers is filled with so much information that he needed days to digest it. But each paper reveals the main message. Our bodies are not responding well to living with so many of the day-to-day fragrances and chemicals that emanate from personal care and cleaning products. We suggest getting a fragrance-chemical divorce in order to start a new, healthier journey through life.

International prevalence of chemical sensitivity, co-prevalences with asthma and autism, and effects from fragrance consumer products

The alarming number of people who report chemical sensitivity, or the fact that autism is a topic of concern as a result of living with chemicals, should be a blaring alarm sound to our government. The study results do not reflect the concern of our government about the current laws that are supposed to be protecting us. The graphs at the end of the article show the alarming numbers of people who are affected by this fragrance-chemical societal explosion. It seems shocking to learn that upwards of 35% of the population has fragrance sensitivity. That would equate to over 100 million people in the United States. That is 1 out of 3 people. Chemical sensitivity for those people reaches as high as 60%. Would the average person change their fragrance habits if they knew they were negatively affecting that percentage of their co-workers, friends, and family? Or will they just casually dismiss their concerns while they fragrance themselves for another attacking day?

Fragranced laundry products and emissions from dryer vents: implications for air quality and health

Most of us have good thoughts about clean laundry. Think again. Learn about the volatile organic compounds (VOCs) in laundry products. How safe is that dryer vent? Does it cause health problems in people? Asthma attacks? Breathing difficulties? Migraine headaches? Is our protective ozone layer negatively impacted by VOCs? Do we understand the chemicals used in these fragranced laundry products? Are dryer vents regulated by any government organization? Dryer vents are like chemical dispersal systems but don't seem to have attracted any attention from lawmakers. Over 12% of the United States general public is negatively affected by scented laundry products. It seems that something most certainly needs to be done to protect those who suffer and those who will.

Volatile Chemical Emissions from Essential Oils with Therapeutic Claims

How about the people who say, "I only use natural oils?" This report concludes that there is toxicity to the wearer, not to mention the intrusiveness on others. Additionally, all of the products end up in our waterways and affect our environment on a large scale.

Pandemic Products and Volatile Chemical Emissions

Most people love a clean house. But when you can smell your neighbor's cleaning products from a hundred yards away, a warning bell in our government's head should sound. This report, similar to the others, reveals that a significant percentage of the population is negatively affected by these products.

The fragranced products phenomenon: air quality and health, science, and policy

We would like the above report to convince people to turn off the volume and flip the light switch off. In other words, our fragrance-free movement encourages people to eliminate the harmful and intrusive fragrances they apply to their skin, use on their clothes, or clean their house with. A manufacturer could use 4,000 ingredients in the composition of one fragrance. There is a prevalence of fragrance sensitivity among the general population. Millions of people are affected negatively by air fresheners. Sensitive people avoid public bathrooms because of them. They affect our health. We believe there are millions of people like us who would vote to work, travel, and dine in a fragrance-free environment. This report details a 35% fragrance sensitivity rate, that 15%-20% report health problems, with disabling health effects reaching much higher, 30%-80% in certain individuals. Loss of workdays and loss of jobs due to fragrance sensitivity range between 6%-15% and the cost is staggering. There are millions of stories of what individuals are inhibited from doing, and what they are missing in their life. Whether this is or isn't the only life we have here on earth, shouldn't people have access to it all without fear of harm around every corner?

<u>Fragrances in the Workplace: what managers need to know</u>

We have highlighted a few comments below from this article above that we thought were powerfully important. This entire research-based article illuminates many of the messages of this book in vivid clarity. It answers questions on fragrance safety. It highlights the changing societal understanding of what fragrances do to others in a negative way, and the cost to society. Pulled from many published studies done by leading experts, and including comparisons of second-hand smoke to the effects of fragrances, it is enlightening information. Begin to understand the magnitude of fragrances' stain on society.

Developing long-lasting fragrance products

The inference is that unscented cosmetics are fragrance-free, which is not always true. The two terms are not interchangeable — which is what smokers found out when they changed to smokeless tobacco.

Unlike tobacco products, some fragrance products are designed to be slow release so that the fragrance dissipates over an extended period of time (Bird, 2008; Fleischer, 2007; and Rosen, 2005;).

Fragrance is a known respiratory irritant and neurological toxin.

Two decades ago, many scientists denied that evidence existed that second-hand smoke was a health hazard and now it is accepted scientific fact. The same change of perspective is happening with Multiple Chemical Sensitivity and synthetic fragrances. Fragrances (containing chemicals) that were thought to have pleasant or neutral effects on health are now acknowledged as either hazardous or potentially hazardous. This is particularly true since chemical formulations of fragrances were changed post WWII with the use of pesticides and petroleum products making fragrance and cleaning products more potent and toxic. The chemicals stay in the air for long periods and can mix and react with other compounds causing additional unknown effects.

Government Entities: If You're Thinking You are Protecting Us, You are Sadly Mistaken

In other words, consumers are the human guinea pigs in this chemical exploding world. Companies are granted enormous leeway when it comes to testing for short-term or long-term illnesses and whether or not certain chemicals are even more dangerous when combined with others. The companies have deep pockets and are swarming with dancing lawyers. The cost and time needed to do the research and testing seems like climbing the unattainable peak of a mountain. But no worries, we've found an elevator to this mountain top, and will talk about it later in this book.

We thought it very important to share some quotes from a meeting way back on October 8, 1985, between the House of Representatives Committee on Science and Technology and the Subcommittee on Investigations and Oversight, Washington, DC. In other words, this was a topic of discussion 37 years ago but the question remains, how much protection are we getting from the government?

The link to this meeting is provided below.

Neurotoxins at Home and in The Workplace

Mr. Harold L. Volkmer, U.S. Representative from Missouri pronounced, "Chemicals are an everyday fact of life in modern society. They enhance our lives in ways too numerous to count, but progress has its price, and too often the price of the role of chemicals in our society is human illness and disease."

Words can be so powerful. But if nothing is done with such powerful words, they just blow into space, where no one hears them. It appears that is the case because synthetic chemicals in the hundreds of thousands are in use today in these staggering amounts in everyday products we use.

He also pointed out that "nerve poisons, called neurotoxins, are one of the leading causes of illness in the workplace. Daily exposure to neurotoxins can cause subtle disorders of the mind and body that cause accidents and injuries. These subtle defects, if undetected and untreated, can lead to irreversible disabling disorders that affect every aspect of the victim's life."

"Neurotoxins are not just an industrial problem. They can be in our children's paint, our perfumes."

Who thinks of neurotoxins as something they should be worried about? Who says, "let's splash, spray and lather on a few neurotoxins in the morning and see what happens?"

From Mr. Don Fuqua, Florida, Chairman

"Recent studies suggest that neurological damage from environmental factors can cause diseases virtually indistinguishable from Parkinson's and Lou Gehrig's disease."

Another U.S. Representative present, Mr. Ronald Packard of California, said, "There are substances commonly used in the home that make our lives easier. We use these substances in good faith, seldom questioning the fact that they could cause peripheral nerve or brain damage."

And from Dr. Bernard Weiss, Toxicology at the University of Rochester, "Not too long ago we viewed the threat of death or serious illness as the main basis on which to control and regulate exposure. Now we also worry about subtle and insidious toxicity expressed mainly as impaired function."

How is it that these comments from 37 years ago didn't resonate louder? It took 40 years after the Toxic Substance Act to revise it. For 40 years, the government sat idle on an Act that wasn't worth the paper it was written on. Why does our government have these hearings if nothing is done after? The comments above should have been an alarm bell to wake the government into action. The headaches, nausea, dizziness, discomfort, difficulty breathing, cancer(s), seem to have been ignored.

We return to the story of the Burn Pits that are sickening our troops across the world. Just yesterday, we came across an old tractor placed in front of a coffee shop. We imagined it burning with its giant rubber tires, steel, foam seats, asbestos, gas running through its core, oil and oil filters, and electronic components, and tried to imagine standing next to it and breathing in that smoke. Then we thought, multiply that tractor times a thousand, add clothes, fragrances and chemicals that make them, guns, ammunition, computers, and most things that come through people's lives and burn it all, breathe it in and imagine, how could it be considered a safe way to dispose of equipment? Yet, Veterans Affairs wants those who are suffering from the ill effects of these Burn Pits to prove, beyond a reasonable doubt, that something else didn't possibly cause their symptoms. There will be more conversation, more requests for testing, more forms to fill out and more delay while Veterans are sick and dying.

After we watched the John Stewart show on these Burn Pits, we had a question. According to the interview, money is not a factor. Why couldn't the government, our military, transport all refuse to a location for safe disposal? Shouldn't we be doing everything possible to protect our troops?

In the 1985 Committee Meeting, Dr. Bernard Weiss also commented that "toxic chemicals are not a new problem. Heavy metals such as mercury and lead have been recognized since antiquity as nervous system poisons."

He goes on to talk about mercury and lead poisons and how they affect brain function and IQ score. He speaks about a major class of workplace chemicals called "volatile organic solvents." He talks about what we should know, but are kept in the dark about.

"Equivalent comments pertain to insecticides. Many of these chemicals are designed specifically to poison the nervous systems of insect pests, so it comes as no surprise that they also can poison the human nervous system.

"Even food additives have been implicated in behavioral toxicity. The Late Ben F. Feingold asserted that many of the children labeled as hyperactive actually were the victims of an elevated sensitivity to certain constituents of the diet, particularly synthetic food colors and flavors.

"Nervous system dysfunction during advanced age seems destined to become the dominant disease entity of the 21st century."

How many years ago was Rachel Carson's *Silent Spring* published about the dangers of pesticides and so much more?

Below is the Statement of Dr. Peter S. Spencer, Director, Institute of Neurotoxicology, Albert Einstein College of Medicine, Bronx, NY:

"I introduce the subject of my discussion with two principles. The first is - The nervous system has an enormous biological responsibility - It allows us to think, remember, recall, to have emotion and personality, to act rationally and responsibly, to sleep and to wake, to walk and to run, to see, smell, taste, hear, and to sense touch and pain.

"Second - The nervous system is commonly affected by chemical substances present in the environment. **Those at greatest risk include the unborn or newborn child whose brain is inadequately shielded from toxic substances in the blood.**

"Other effects of environmental chemicals are long-lasting, permanent, and sometimes even progressive. Such changes may occur with single or repeated chemical insult to the nervous system.

"Hundreds of other compounds used in fragrance formulations remain to be tested for chronic neurobehavioral toxicity.

"We are ignorant to the long-term effects of substances with neurotoxic potential added to food, present in skin care products, or used in the workplace."

Another concern brought up by the Committee was that "The neurological community, in particular, was incredibly surprised to learn of the possible association between chemical exposure and Parkinsonism.

"Now, suddenly, with this new awareness, the neurological community is beginning to ask questions about other disorders such as Lou Gehrig's disease and Alzheimer's disease. Could this possibly be the result of chemical exposure?"

We repeat Dr. Peter S. Spencer's quotes above to prove without a doubt that what is going on in the fragrance and personal care industry, the chemicals used and the harm to us, the human population, is an experiment worthy of a horror movie where all life is a gigantic experiment run by greed and profit, and where all life is systematically slowly being eliminated. Those in the fragrance and chemical industries and the government will continue to request more testing at a snail's pace while these chemicals are free to roam through our bodies.

Other quotes from Dr. Weiss at the same hearing are: "The risk of lung cancer is elevated in asbestos workers. The risk of lung cancer is elevated in people who smoke. Combine the two and the elevation is just enormous. Only recently has our consciousness about mixtures been raised because it's dawned on everybody that, unlike the laboratory, the real world exposes us to enormous numbers of substances all at once."

That this comment is made at this hearing in the year 1985 shows how unbelievably we've been taken advantage of as "test subjects." Furthermore, it continues today with more chemicals that aren't tested, haven't been tested and most likely won't be tested. Let's just say it, the substances in use have not been tested alone or in combination with two others or with hundreds of others. Our "Intrusive Potion #21" fragrance-chemical punch bowl is all the evidence anyone needs to know about what chemicals are in that bowl and how they are reacting with one another. It is a noxious mixture.

We are using part of this same transcript, as each person quoted below has had invaluable information to share and we thought it important to add clarity to this book's messages.

From Don R. Clay, Director, U.S. Environmental Protection Agency in the year 1985.

"The Toxic Substance Control Act (TSCA) is a risk-balancing statute. It requires the EPA to carefully consider the economic impacts of its decisions, including whether they unduly impede or create unnecessary barriers to technological innovation. Risk-benefit analysis is a complex and difficult process, but it is inherent in every decision made under TSCA, Toxic Substance Control Act." In other words, progress trumps individuals' rights for a safe environment.

"There are over 850 known neurotoxic chemicals, as pointed out by Anger & Johnson."

Dr. McMillan

"As Mr. Clay has stated, there are approximately 8 million known chemicals. Recently, a select committee of the National Academy of Sciences identified somewhere in excess of 50,000 of those chemicals where human exposure is likely. Nor does it include any one of the tremendously large number of mixtures of chemical compounds."

This mixture of chemicals is exactly what we breathe every day, without knowledge of its health effects on us. When you take into account 50,000 chemicals or today it's above 80,000 and rising fast, the combinations explode in size and scope. It is inconceivable to expect our government to do testing on these 80,000 let alone combinations of two or hundreds that will exceed the millions and millions and millions. "Overwhelming" or "that which will be avoided" will lead us into darkness.

Toxic Substances Control Act of 1976

The Toxic Substances Control Act (TSCA or TOSCA) is a United States law, passed by the 94th United States Congress in 1976 and administered by the United States Environmental Protection Agency (EPA), that regulates the introduction of new or already existing chemicals. When the TSCA was put into place, almost all existing chemicals were considered to be safe for use and subsequently grandfathered in. In other words, the EPA has not been protecting us as well as we might like.

The links below show the enormous complexity in determining the dangers of each chemical. These Acts talk about the processes involved in evaluating safety and the guidelines to be even considered a candidate for regulation or testing.

Summary of the Toxic Substances Control Act -

Frank R. Lautenberg Chemical Safety for the 21st Century Act, which updates the Toxic Substances Control Act

The Frank R. Lautenberg Chemical Safety for the 21st Century Act Implementation Activities

For the First Time in 40 Years EPA to Put in Place a Process to Evaluate Chemicals that May Pose Risk

Prioritizing Existing Chemicals for Risk Evaluation complex at the least

TSCA mandates timelines for both prioritization and risk evaluation. Prioritization must take between 9 and 12 months (Section 6(b)(2)(C)) and risk evaluation must be completed within three years, with a potential six-month extension. Considering the chemicals that need testing, and new untested chemicals flooding the market, in whose lifetime are people going to be safe from toxic chemicals?

TSCA Work Plan for Chemical Assessments: 2014 Update

If you read about the Toxic Substance Control Act and the new Frank R. Lautenberg Chemical Safety for the 21st Century Act and the other links provided, it's hard to not worry about back doors, side doors, hidden doors, and other escape hatches to exclude a chemical from safety testing. This is an overwhelming amount of information to read, digest, or even care about. It would be so easy to throw up your arms and say, "Whatever. I'll take my chances on the chemicals in my products." We completely understand that stance. But to realize now that the dangers were first considered 40 years ago and we are yet to be protected, should be enough to make anyone pause. Does anyone have the right to choose their personal care products and use them as they please, without consideration for the health and well-being of others? It seems to mimic the COVID mask and vaccine debate raging in our country right now. What about the common good?

The Environmental Defense Fund - A Primer on the New Toxic Substance Control Act and what led to it, highlights the first act and all the escape hatches. Here, we learned how much influence the chemical manufacturing industry and environmental groups had in drafting the first Act and less of an influence drafting the new law. There are **lines of text in this new control Act that might nullify, eliminate**

and/or neutralize, the power of the Act. In other words, being protected by government is still highly questionable.

Our government has avoided the mountain of chemicals in commerce and how to stop it from growing. They have yet to solve how to reasonably get the correct data required in an expeditious manner and how to remove what has existed in the products we have used for decades now without loss of jobs. They do not know how to stop all the new chemicals from entering the commerce arena without first testing. So, we are safe?

The FDA

The FDA is separate from the EPA in its responsibilities.

Fragrances in Cosmetics

Who is responsible for substantiating the safety of cosmetics?

"Companies and individuals who manufacture or market cosmetics have a legal responsibility to ensure the safety of their products," which is also known as "self-regulation" and is a very troubling matter.

Does the FDA approve cosmetics before they go on the market?

"FDA's legal authority over cosmetics is different from our authority over other products we regulate, such as drugs, biologics, and medical devices. Under the law, cosmetic products and ingredients do not need FDA premarket approval." And the FDA thinks they are protecting us how?

Just like the EPA, holes seem to be plentiful in "protection under the FDA rule of law." Some of the data supplied in the links in this book tell stories worth reading about the chemicals and fragrances in the cosmetic world. Your face, your beautiful face. Protect it!

FDA Authority Over Cosmetics: How Cosmetics Are Not FDA-Approved, but Are FDA-Regulated

Cosmetics & U.S. Law

A Temporary Solution Suggestion

To avoid the fragrance laws that aren't protecting us until we put together an army of lawyers ready to fight on our behalf, let's let all fragranced products lie dead on shelves as the first step to immediate change. We have the choice, an absolute right, to choose to not use fragranced products. We don't need the fragrance and chemical industries' permission to do anything. Nor do we need to listen to them. We have heard loud and clear that the chemicals they use in our products, for years and years, have not been deemed safe. We are hoping to get more people to make the fragrance-free choice and to "Turn Yourself Off."

Ultimate Thoughts

WHY IN 1976 DID CONGRESS FINALLY decide we needed a Toxic Substance Control Act? How were they watching our backs all those years before?

How many of the thousands of chemicals that Congress was "worried about" when they passed the 1976 law were grandfathered in?

As a person is lying in a hospital surgery room with their vital organs exposed, how safe is it that hundreds of chemicals have the opportunity to attach to those organs and reach into their bloodstream from the fragranced products that are coming off the medical assistants and/or surgeons who shouldn't be wearing fragranced products, but just might be?

It seems inconceivable that retail stores can pollute the air with fragrances and chemicals out the front door in overpowering amounts of smell strength and chemical load, with no government intervention.

Some people want to know their body burden score. They can learn the score in the game they are playing against the invisible enemy, chemicals in fragranced products.

Asking manufacturers to police and self-regulate their actions is as ridiculous as asking society to police itself and eliminate the police force.

Is it possible that your allergies / asthma would improve without chemicals on your face and body? Why not give it a try? Aim to stop breathing in chemicals all day, every day. Try just breathing in chemically free air. We are confident you will feel amazing.

Even at 9/11 Ground Zero, the exact cause of all those cancers is still in question. What isn't in question are the chemicals of concern in the toxic cloud of dust. Why continue to take chances on using products made with the same chemicals in question from 9/11? Don't be a guinea pig to the chemical world. Why live in a 9/11 toxic cloud of uncertainty?

If you want to know what deception looks like, read this 9/11 report. How many of the chemicals in the fragranced products used by billions play a part in the game of deception? After reading this report and the links provided, we find it impossible to place our health in the hands of the EPA. We believe you will feel the same.

"Stronger, longer lasting, more powerful." These are the words of the fragrance industry. What is the end goal? Fragrances contain phthalates, fixatives and plasticizers, chemicals that help fragrances last longer but that have been clearly proven to cause a long list of human ailments. The links provided in this book contain our research sources and are full of stories about the health risks of these chemicals, which manufacturers do not have to list under "Ingredients." We say it again, "Why live in a 9/11 toxic cloud of uncertainty? And why bring a 9/11 toxic cloud of uncertainty with you everywhere you go and subject others to the same?"

For those who can't stand the smell of their own work clothes at the end of the day and rely on super fragranced products to eliminate it, try washing in hot water with baking soda and afterwards letting them hang outside to air out. Don't add a new fragrance that millions say affects them negatively to replace work clothes smell. Let hot water, baking soda, and time be the chemical-free natural course to choose.

For many years now we have the habit of dipping our faces in ice water to refresh our face skin naturally each morning. But trying to hold his breath for more than a minute, is the "best Bob can do." It reminds him that lack of air brings him close to death. Without air to breathe, we die. We are appealing for more clean air to breathe. Fragrance- and chemical-free air.

We believe that clean, breathable air is a basic human right.

Thank you!

What Scent them Away?

Take me back to 1962 when DDT snow fell in the Silent Spring
Eyes read, but ears turned away
As we watched in silent expression as Robins sang
With questions we didn't comprehend, and no answers
Robins fell in that snowy silent spring

I wake each day with a voice I say
Why did you leave me, what scent you away?
I loved you dear, you, my wife.
Why did you leave me, what scent you away?
Will the world's synthetic hand
Send us all away
I loved you dear
Never to be taken away
I can smell you still
Sadly, I always will

Chemicals of concern
A list of more than many
I'm here to say
Don't go away
Names are long
In moonlight or under the clouds that play
Whom do we point fingers at to say?
What were you thinking?

Persistent organic pollutants
Don't go away

As we all lay loved ones to rest
They forgot to say, we didn't test
Not in combinations of two or many
Why bother, times on our side, before truths come clear
In my Ivory tower, I hold so dear
Because of the money you spend
My life will be merry until the very end

As for suffering, we've seen it in you
Yeah, little government protection, you can't see, but we're laughing at you
You, our Guinea Pigs, have and always will be
You're not smart enough to stay away
And until that time comes
Who's to say, a millennium of moons away
I'll live in my Ivory tower
You can all just die away

The World Trade Center exploded in a chemical cloud of dust
Those covered in dust
With no one to trust
Most are sick or died away
With generations to follow
It's hard to swallow
They didn't see it coming
But here's the rub, others knew that first day
Toxic chemicals just don't fly away

Our human genes became homes to stay
Those generations to follow
We all feel your sorrow

As we remember that chemical cloud of dust

9/11 that clear sky day

It most certainly didn't fly away

Opposite of what they told you

Help us anyway

Then, we don't care, just die away

Stop the crying in hospital rooms that soar high above

Please don't take the children away

Smiles that light up skies

Are flying to heaven too early

All that have lost, say

What were you thinking?

What scent them away?

Hyperlinks

350,000 synthetic chemicals - https://apple.news/AzPesDr3gQBiGvyFa-bZJpg

Agent Orange - https://en.wikipedia.org/wiki/Agent_Orange

Asbestos - https://en.wikipedia.org/wiki/Asbestos

DDT - https://www.epa.gov/ingredients-used-pesticide-products/ddt-brief-history-and-status

Lead Paint - https://en.wikipedia.org/wiki/Lead_paint

Cigarette Smoke - https://www.cdc.gov/tobacco/data_statistics/fact_sheets/health_effects/effects_cig_smoking/index.htm

Low-Level Chemical Exposure: A Challenge for Science and Policy - https://dspace.mit.edu/bitstream/handle/1721.1/115577/es983778h.pdf?sequence=1

Fragrance: emerging health and environmental concerns - https://onlinelibrary.wiley.com/doi/epdf/10.1002/ffj.1106

Nuclear Power in the World Today - https://world-nuclear.org/information-library/current-and-future-generation/nuclear-power-in-the-world-today.aspx

Cancer Alley - https://www.propublica.org/article/welcome-to-cancer-alley-where-toxic-air-is-about-to-get-worse

How the heart works - https://www.hoag.org/specialties-services/heart-vascular/conditions/heart-basics/

Menstrual cycle: What's normal, what's not - https://www.mayoclinic.org/healthy-lifestyle/womens-health/in-depth/menstrual-cycle/art-20047186

12 systems of the body - https://hunterbusinessschool.edu/medical-assistant-program-diploma-training-body-systems-disorders/

Olfactory Fatigue - https://en.wikipedia.org/wiki/Olfactory_fatigue

The sense of smell - https://www.niehs.nih.gov/news/events/pastmtg/hazmat/assets/2012/6_sense_of_smell_508.pdf

Hyperosmia - https://en.wikipedia.org/wiki/Hyperosmia

Biosphere 2 - https://www.bizjournals.com/bizwomen/news/profiles-strategies/2015/02/jane-poynter-spent-two-years-in-a-3-acre-dome-when.html?page=all

Considered Chemistry at Nike - https://greenchemistryandcommerce.org/downloads/Nike_final.pdf

Harmful Chemicals in Tobacco Products - https://www.cancer.org/cancer/cancer-causes/tobacco-and-cancer/carcinogens-found-in-tobacco-products.html

The Four Dog Defense - https://aesm.assembly.ca.gov/sites/aesm.assembly.ca.gov/files/The%20Four%20Dog%20Defense%20with%20pics.pdf

Copy of a Study of Cigarette Advertising Made By J.W. Burgard, 1953 - https://www.industrydocuments.ucsf.edu/tobacco/docs/#id=qymm0104

A Study of People's Cigarette Smoking Habits and Attitudes - https://www.industrydocuments.ucsf.edu/tobacco/docs/#id=qjjb0040

International prevalence of chemical sensitivity, co-prevalences with asthma and autism, and effects from fragrance consumer products - https://link.springer.com/article/10.1007/s11869-019-00672-1. Or should I use this: https://rdcu.be/cFMHx

Fragranced laundry products and emissions from dryer vents: implications for air quality and health - https://researchonline.jcu.edu.au/64706/1/JCU_64706.pdf

Volatile Chemical Emissions from Essential Oils with Therapeutic Claims - https://researchonline.jcu.edu.au/64707/2/JCU_64707_accepted.pdf

Pandemic Products and Volatile Chemical Emissions - https://researchonline.jcu.edu.au/64449/2/JCU_64449_Steinemann2021_accepted.pdf

The fragranced products phenomenon: air quality and health, science and policy - https://researchonline.jcu.edu.au/64708/1/64708.pdf

Fragrances in the Workplace: what managers need to know - https://www.renevanmaarsseveen.nl/wp-content/uploads/overig5/Geur%20-%20wat%20managers%20moeten%20weten%20(EN).pdf

Neurotoxins at Home and in The Workplace - Neurotoxins at Home and in The Workplace

Toxic Substances Control Act of 1976 - https://en.wikipedia.org/wiki/Toxic_Substances_Control_Act_of_1976

Summary of the Toxic Substances Control Act - https://www.epa.gov/laws-regulations/summary-toxic-substances-control-act

Frank R. Lautenberg Chemical Safety for the 21st Century Act, which updates the Toxic Substances Control Act - https://www.epa.gov/assessing-and-managing-chemicals-under-tsca/frank-r-lautenberg-chemical-safety-21st-century-act

The Frank R. Lautenberg Chemical Safety for the 21st Century Act Implementation Activities - https://www.epa.gov/assessing-and-managing-chemicals-under-tsca/frank-r-lautenberg-chemical-safety-21st-century-act-4

For the First Time in 40 Years EPA to Put in Place a Process to Evaluate Chemicals that May Pose Risk - https://archive.epa.gov/epa/newsreleases/first-time-40-years-epa-put-place-process-evaluate-chemicals-may-pose-risk.html

Prioritizing Existing Chemicals for Risk Evaluation complex at the least - https://www.epa.gov/assessing-and-managing-chemicals-under-tsca/prioritizing-existing-chemicals-risk-evaluation

TSCA Work Plan for Chemical Assessments: 2014 Update - https://www.epa.gov/sites/default/files/2015-01/documents/tsca_work_plan_chemicals_2014_update-final.pdf

Environmental Defense Fund - A Primer on the New Toxic Substance Control Act and what led to it - https://www.edf.org/sites/default/files/denison-primer-on-lautenberg-act.pdf

Fragrances in Cosmetics - https://www.fda.gov/cosmetics/cosmetic-ingredients/fragrances-cosmetics#how

FDA Authority Over Cosmetics: How Cosmetics Are Not FDA-Approved, but Are FDA-Regulated - https://www.fda.gov/cosmetics/cosmetics-laws-regulations/fda-authority-over-cosmetics-how-cosmetics-are-not-fda-approved-are-fda-regulated

Cosmetics & U.S. Law - https://www.fda.gov/cosmetics/cosmetics-laws-regulations/cosmetics-us-law#Assuring_Ingredient_and_Product_Safety

9/11 - https://en.wikipedia.org/wiki/Health_effects_arising_from_the_September_11_attacks

We live a
fragrance-free
lifestyle

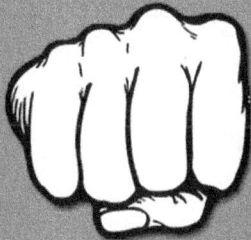

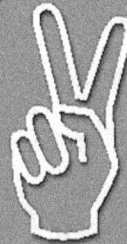

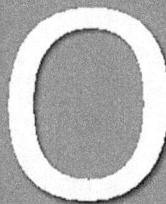

Fist bumps &
virtual hugs
please

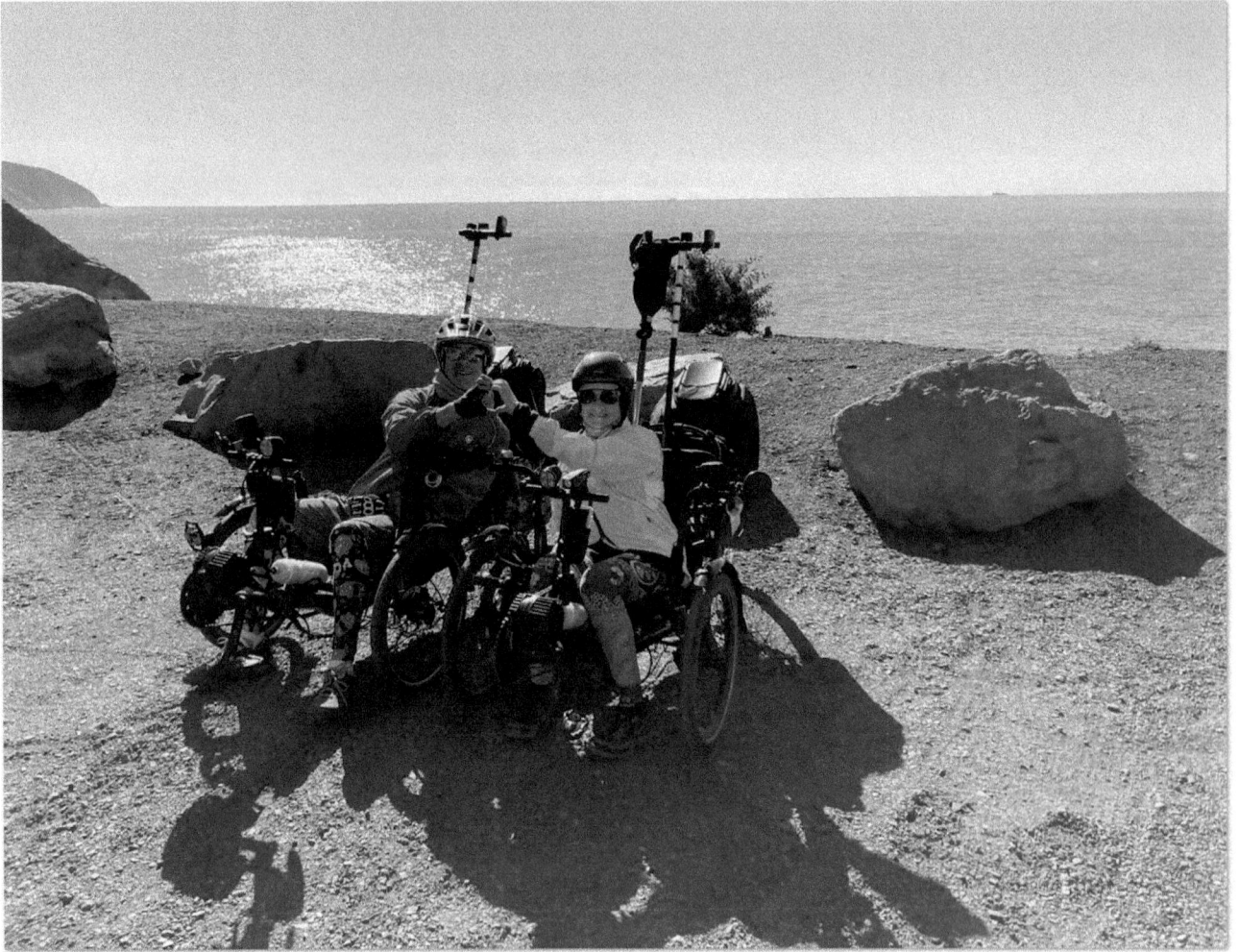

Thank You!

www.ingramcontent.com/pod-product-compliance
Lightning Source LLC
Chambersburg PA
CBHW080802300326
41914CB00055B/1019